Sarah Chaney is a research fellow at the Queen Mary Centre for the History of the Emotions. She spent her teens and twenties furiously rebelling against the mainstream, whilst secretly longing to be normal. It wasn't until she passed thirty that she (mostly) stopped worrying about this mythical ideal. Alongside her research work she runs the public exhibitions and events programme at the Royal College of Nursing, and reads far too much X-Men fanfic.

Praise for *Am I Normal?*

'Eureka! Sarah Chaney's excellent *Am I Normal?* is one of those rare pop-science books that make you look at the whole world differently' *Daily Telegraph* ★★★★★

'Captivating' Book of the Day, *Guardian*

'Compelling, highly readable … Encompassing everything from sex surveys to baby weight, beauty standards to sexuality, this is a brilliantly engaging work of popular science' *Observer*

'Sarah Chaney charts, fascinatingly, [a] progressive creep of the idea of the "normal" into the heart of society … shocking and salutary' *The Times*

'Riveting … The moral of the story, indeed of this engaging book, is that instead of ruminating endlessly on the worried (and unanswerable) question 'am I normal?', we should be asking ourselves instead whether normal even exists and why, quite frankly, anyone cares' *Mail on Sunday* ★★★★★

'This fascinating read will change the way we think about what is normal' *Buzz*

**wellcome
collection**

Wellcome Collection publishes thought-provoking books exploring health and human experience, in partnership with leading independent publisher Profile Books.

Wellcome Collection is a free museum and library that aims to challenge how we think and feel about health by connecting science, medicine, life and art, through exhibitions, collections, live programming, and more. It is part of Wellcome, a global charitable foundation that supports science to solve urgent health challenges, with a focus on mental health, infectious diseases and climate.

wellcomecollection.org

AM I NORMAL?

THE 200-YEAR SEARCH FOR NORMAL PEOPLE

(And Why They Don't Exist)

SARAH CHANEY

P

PROFILE BOOKS

wellcome
collection

This paperback edition published in 2023

First published in Great Britain in 2022 by
Profile Books Ltd
29 Cloth Fair
London
ECIA 7JQ
www.profilebooks.com

Published in association with Wellcome Collection

183 Euston Road
London NWI 2BE
www.wellcomecollection.org

Text design by James Alexander/Jade Design

1 3 5 7 9 10 8 6 4 2

Printed and bound in Great Britain by
CPI Group (UK) Ltd, Croydon CRO 4YY

A CIP catalogue record for this book is available from the British Library.

ISBN 978 1 78816 246 3
eISBN 978 1 78283 544 8

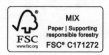

For Sadie and Willow, who are both too
remarkable to ever merely be normal.

CONTENTS

A NOTE ON THE SURVEYS AND QUESTIONNAIRES

To underscore the questions posed in this book, you'll find a selection of original historical questionnaires from the nineteenth and twentieth centuries reproduced between pages 272 and 284: from the 1889 Census of Hallucinations to Mass Observation's 1949 sex survey. These documents were used by doctors, scientists and sociologists to try to pinpoint where the normal might lie in relation to the body, mind, feelings and sex lives of their fellow humans. Nothing, perhaps, better shows how elusive and mutable the idea of what's normal really is. Have a go and embrace your 'failure' to fit the normal standard.

PROLOGUE
AM I NORMAL?

It seems like a straightforward enough question, on the face of it. It's something you might ask yourself on a regular basis. Is my body a normal shape or size? Is it normal to cry in front of others? To let my dog lick my face? To have heavy periods? To have sex with strangers? To feel anxious on public transport? To feel bloated after eating? These and countless other questions frame and explain our lives. They help us negotiate our relationships with other people and work out when we might need intervention: the advice of a friend or a visit to the doctor.

They also prove how complex the idea of normality is.

What do we mean when we ask if we're normal? Even just taking the questions in the paragraph above, this varies enormously. Sometimes we're considering if we're more or less average – or perhaps slightly above or below average, if that seems more socially desirable. I might want to be a little above average height, for example, and a little below average weight.

On other occasions, we're wondering if we're healthy. Is my blood pressure normal? If I feel pain in a certain place, is it a sign that something is medically wrong? If your child sleepwalks, this might be classed as normal not because it's common (a 2004 Sleep in America Poll found that just 2 per cent of school-aged children sleepwalk several nights a week or more) but because it's not considered unhealthy.

Most often, however, when we ask if we're normal we're wondering if we're like other people. Am I a typical example of the human race? Do I react in the same way as other people to situations? Do I look or dress or talk like other people? If I was *more* like them, would my life be easier?

These questions can have profound effects on our lives. I was a shy and awkward child, with thick plastic-rimmed NHS glasses and much-loved home-knitted jumpers, who spent most of her time buried in books dreaming of a better, more magical world. By the start of secondary school in the early 1990s, I was already marked out as abnormal, for reasons best known to my peers. 'Creepy Phoebe', they used to call me, after the bespectacled teenage *Neighbours* character, whose father was a funeral director and scared her classmates by keeping pet snakes. By the age of sixteen I was a ball of barely contained fury at the world, spending most of the school day wearing headphones so that no one would talk to me while I scratched Manic Street Preachers lyrics across every wooden school desk.

Does any of this sound familiar? If so, perhaps I was a normal teenager after all. But, like most teens, I never *felt* normal. As many bullied young people do, I accepted the outcast label that was handed to me and took it as my own (or so I thought), stubbornly exaggerating those differences my bullies commented on to distance myself from them still further. It was stupid, I thought, for there to be a rule that wearing a backpack on both shoulders or pulling your socks up to keep your legs warm was 'square', so I insisted on doing both. I didn't want to wear make-up and listen to pop music but to spend every glorious Wednesday with my head buried in the new issue of *NME* or *Melody Maker* reading about bands no one else in my school had even heard of.

Despite all this, there was a part of me that longed to be normal. If one of the bands I liked made the top ten, I felt like I'd achieved something – other people liked something I did! The normal was a mysteriously vague ideal that stayed with me throughout early adulthood, brought into sharp relief by a dread of not fitting in, a fear of being abandoned and alone, and a sense that if something magically changed in or about me then everything would suddenly be okay. I was probably approaching thirty before I really questioned what I meant by 'being normal'.

If you've picked up this book, it's probably because you've had similar fears, or asked yourself similar questions. So, is a dread of being different actually normal? Have people always worried about attaining a particular set of life goals in this way? When do we embrace our differences from other people and when do we fear them? And who gets to decide what's normal anyway?

In what follows, I reveal how short the history of worrying about being normal really is. Of course, in some circumstances people have always judged themselves by those around them or criticised others for not fitting in.

However, it was only in the last 200 years that this began to happen on a widespread scale, enshrined in scientific practice in Europe and North America through medicine, physiology, psychology, sociology and criminology – driven by the rapid rise of statistics. Normality became bound up in our laws, our social structures, and our ideas of health. But before 1800, the word 'normal' was not even associated with human behaviour at all. Normal was a mathematical term, referring to a right angle.

The growing popularity of statistics in Europe and North America in the nineteenth century inspired scientists to measure humanity to find first an average, and then a norm. These norms could not have been set without the standardisation of huge swathes of human life that defined what and who was normal – and by implication most human, most valuable. The introduction of compulsory education in many countries, for example, led to the identification of children who learned more slowly than their classmates, while the creation of national insurance and occupational compensation schemes demanded medical screening with increasingly detailed definitions of normal health. Baby-weighing clinics gave rise to enduring ideas about childhood development, IQ tests began to establish norms of intelligence, and factories and industrial workplaces gave rise to notions of the ideal worker and standard productivity levels. Colonial expansion by Western countries sent scientists out to measure and define around the globe, comparing the population of their own homelands with people elsewhere – almost always in ways that favoured white people. This book focuses on Europe and North America simply because that was where the so-called normal was born: the assumption that these standards applied to the rest of the world was just that, an assumption.

The science of the normal these researchers created, then, is also a story about the othering of whole communities, defined in opposition to Western standards of the 'right' way for a person to be. The scientists, doctors and scholars who attempted to measure and standardise humanity were overwhelmingly white, wealthy, Western men, who were exclusively heterosexual (at least in public). They tended to support the status quo – which they had to thank for their success – and marginalise other groups in the process. When they desired change, it was most often change that benefitted their educated professional class. This is not to say that this was always intentional or that none of these men ever supported those less privileged. Some called themselves socialists; others backed the feminist movement, denounced imperial aggression, or argued that homosexuality should be legalised.

Yet most of these men also assumed that their place at the top of the social ladder was simply the natural order of things. They had been born into the highest stage of human evolution – or so they believed – and charitably sought to set a standard to help others improve. One of the arguments made at the time to justify colonialism was that the lives of the peoples colonised were improved by being guided in Western norms – or rather, as we might put it today, by having Western norms brutally enforced upon them. In India, for example, hundreds of thousands of people were killed by British troops, and millions more died in recurrent famines as the British government exported Indian goods for commercial gain. Meanwhile, in Indian public schools, colonial teachers proudly described how they created 'real' – or normal – boys, defined in the image of their colonisers through the adoption of British sports and dress.[1] In the US, it was Federal policy to 'acculturate and assimilate' indigenous people 'by eradicating their tribal cultures through a boarding school system' until 1934.[2] Whereas, in the seventeenth and eighteenth centuries, many colonial governments had maintained a distance between their subjects and those of the countries they colonised, as the nineteenth century progressed normalisation became central to colonial rule.

Such examples from the past can seem dramatically and obviously wrong to us today. But is it merely a sobering thought to recall how many people have been killed, imprisoned, ruled insane or otherwise excluded from society because of the shifting notion of what's normal? Or is there something more we can take from this history? I believe there is. Although we constantly refine and expand our definitions of what is normal, natural or desirable, many of us never stop to consider if there is such a thing at all. We just assume the normal exists, an invisible law of nature – perhaps slightly to the left or right of where our parents or our grandparents told us it was, but there nonetheless.

Yet this so-called normal may not even be all that usual. In 2010, three North American behavioural scientists suggested that the sub-section of the world's population from which today's scientific norms are drawn – which differs surprisingly little from the groups studied by nineteenth-century scientists – might be the 'WEIRDest people

6

in the world'. People from WEIRD (that is, Western, educated, industrialised, rich and democratic) societies make
up just 12 per cent of the world's population but 96 per
cent of subjects in psychology studies and 80 per cent in
medicine.[3] They are assumed to be white – even when they
are not – because white is supposed to be a neutral category
as far as science and medicine is concerned.[4] The Victorian
science of the 'normal' has a long legacy.

But when drugs and treatments are designed for WEIRD
(and white, and male) people, how can we expect them
to offer the best outcomes for everybody else?[5] Diseases
show up differently in men and women, or in people with
different skin tones. Until 1990, it was common for drugs
to be tested only on men – it was cheaper and easier for
researchers, because men's hormone levels don't tend to
fluctuate, as is the case for many women. The problem
was that, once on the market, these drugs and treatments
weren't always suitable for the women taking them. Dr
Alyson McGregor's *Sex Matters* describes how prescription
medications may be withdrawn from the US market due to
unexpected side effects in women. It wasn't, for example,
until after sleep aid Ambien had become widely available
that the dose for women was halved, when it was realised
that women tend to metabolise the drug at a slower rate
than men.[6] These women woke up drowsier, the drug still
in their systems during a potentially unsafe drive to work.
But why hadn't this been discovered sooner?

While some scientists 'routinely assume' that findings
from WEIRD studies can be generalised to the other 88 per
cent of the world's population, others have claimed that
WEIRD people may be 'among the least representative

populations one could find for generalizing about humans'.[7] So how has our history led us to a position where such a tiny group continues to dominate narratives of what it is to be 'normal'?

By exploring the history of the contested ways in which norms and standards have been adopted I hope to encourage you to question not only what you think of as normal, but also why we are so ready to define ourselves by such prescriptive judgements. I invite you to consider how the 'normal' permeates our lives and the impact it has on us, whether you are WEIRD or not. If, like most people, you have ever feared being different, I hope you will find this book thought-provoking and liberating.

It may be normal to worry about being normal. But that shouldn't stop us questioning the very idea.

1

A BRIEF HISTORY
OF THE NORMAL

NATURE'S ERRORS

The story of the normal as we know it begins on New Year's Day 1801, with an Italian priest and astronomer, Giuseppe Piazzi. He spotted a new star in the sky while searching for a planet between Mars and Jupiter. Piazzi tracked the movements of this star – which he named Ceres after the Roman goddess of agriculture – until 11 February, when it was too close to the sun and disappeared. In October (news travelled considerably more slowly in those pre-internet days) Piazzi's published data reached the twenty-four-year-old German mathematician Carl Friedrich Gauss.

Whereas Piazzi had been unable to take enough measurements to determine Ceres' orbit, Gauss used a mathematical formula to create an average that, when plotted on a graph, created a rough bell-shaped curve, rising into a rounded peak at the centre with a long tail on either side. Gauss claimed that Ceres would emerge at the point shown in the exact centre of this curve. On the next clear night, the young mathematician was proven right. The German star spotter's name soon became associated with the bell curve and even today it is sometimes known as a Gaussian distribution.* At first, however, it was called the 'error curve'.[1]

For centuries, astronomers had recognised that measurements in their field were subject to mistakes. They accounted for this by taking a large number of measurements. Small errors were made more often than large ones, and it was this that created the shape of the curve plotted by Gauss. So far, so good. You might have done a very basic version of this yourself when putting up shelves or something. Checking measurements over and over before drilling the necessary holes. I'm invariably a few millimetres out, all the same. But what on earth do the efforts of astronomers – and amateur carpenters – to accurately measure distance have to do with the norms of human life?

We owe the collision to one very active Belgian statistician: Adolphe Quetelet, born in Ghent in 1796. There's a street named after this scientist in Brussels, where the former royal observatory – Quetelet's home for forty years – was located. I visited a few years ago, and charity workers in the former observatory building no doubt wondered why someone was taking photos of their office. Place Quetelet was just an ordinary city street. Unremarkable. Normal. Quetelet, who idealised the ordinary, would probably have been happy with this development.

The young Adolphe Quetelet grew up in a turbulent

* Or a Gauss–Laplace distribution, by those who also credit the French mathematician Pierre-Simon Laplace, who proposed using an error curve to predict the outcome of an event nearly thirty years earlier.

time for Belgium, which drove his passion for understanding human society. Ghent was controlled by Napoleonic France during his childhood but then, when the statistician was nineteen years old, the Dutch-speaking city became part of the United Kingdom of the Netherlands, and he studied science at the newly founded University of Ghent. Then, in 1830, the Belgian Revolution came along and cast his young career as royal astronomer into disarray – the observatory was very nearly turned into an arsenal.[2] The revolution sent Quetelet on a path away from astronomy to the study of society: he brought with him, however, the astronomer's methods.

In 1835, five years after the revolution, Quetelet published his most famous book: *On Man and the Development of His Faculties, or Essay on Social Physics.*[3] Seeking order in human society after the recent upheaval, Quetelet took the astronomer's error curve and applied it to human measurements. It was not obvious this would work, given the significant difference in the kinds of data. Pinpointing a star's correct location is not the same as, say, measuring human height. There is no 'true' measurement of height, only an average based on the most common height in a population. It's important to remember, however, that the background of truth and error in astronomy meant that the normal in humans was, from the very first, bound up in the assumption that the normal was *correct*, as well as average. Those people who did not meet the normal ideal became errors – not, this time, of the astronomer, but mistakes of God or nature.

One simple graph, then, began the scientific obsession with the normal. The bell curve remains in widespread use

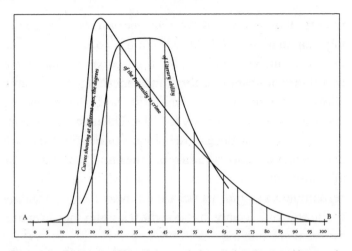

Curves showing at different ages, the degrees

of the propensity to crime

of literary ability

A

B

0   5   10   15   20   25   30   35   40   45   50   55   60   65   70   75   80   85   90   95   100

A chart from Quetelet's 1835 book on social physics, showing a roughly normal distribution (of literary ability in the population) and a rather more skewed curve, supposedly detailing the propensity to crime at different ages.

across the social and life sciences today; you might dimly remember it from school. But its origin makes it clear how far the normal distribution has diverged from its intended function. There are many things that affect human measurements that don't apply to the location of stars, after all. Take height. In the UK, Mr Average stands at 5 foot 9, while Ms Average is 5 foot 3.5.[4] Around 95 per cent of the adult population is within two standard deviations of this height: that is, between 5 foot 4 and 6 foot 1 for men and 4 foot 11 and 5 foot 8 for women. Of course, 95 per cent of the population isn't even *nearly* everyone. More than 3 million people in Britain fall outside these parameters: that's more than the total population of Barbados, Brunei, Djibouti, Luxembourg and Malta combined. And what of Mx Average? Anyone gender-fluid or non-binary simply disappears from such studies; just the first example of how normal statistics can and do privilege certain ways of defining a population.

The limits and shape of the bell curve can also alter depending on the group being measured. If we combined all sexes on one scale, we'd get a different result.[*5] Taking ethnicity or age into account will also change things. And then there's gravity: our measurements will differ slightly if taken when we first wake up, or at the end of the day. After all, astronauts can gain up to 2 inches while in orbit, as the vertebrae in the spine expand and relax.

It quickly becomes clear that a seemingly factual measure like normal height is less straightforward than it first appears. Despite this, the bell curve is still in regular use as a way of summing up the characteristics of a population – though its creators peering through telescopes never dreamed of it as a measure of human attributes, let alone as a yardstick of normality.

THE AVERAGE MAN

So how and why did people start to think of themselves as 'normal'? Before about 1820, the word normal was not used by anyone to describe themselves or each other; nor was it used by scientists or doctors to understand human populations. Normal was a term used in maths, for angles, equations and formulae. People weren't normal: lines and calculations were.

* You might assume that this would lead to a graph with two distinct peaks (a bimodal distribution). However, if you have a large sample of people, it often instead results in a differently shaped normal distribution.

There were, perhaps, some hints that the meaning of normal was already changing. When I visited Ghent a few years ago, in pursuit of the early science of the normal, I found myself staying just off Normaalschoolstraat. Of course, I took a selfie with the street sign. The first 'Normal School' was opened in Vienna in 1771, followed two decades later by the most famous, the École Normale in Paris. These schools were seen as models of exemplary education, though in continental Europe and the US today, normal school usually refers to a teacher training school. The town of Normal, Illinois, was named in 1865 after the teacher training college located there. The same is true of most other towns called Normal – there are four in the US alone. The notion that graduates of normal schools might embody a desirable model for shaping the younger generation began to nudge the meaning of the word towards its later definition.

Quetelet's great concept was that of the 'average man' (or *l'homme moyenne*). Based on his statistical analysis, he thought the average man was the truest representation of humanity. While we might scorn mediocrity, to Quetelet to be average was to be perfect. 'Every quality, taken within suitable limits, is essentially good,' Quetelet professed; 'it is only in its extreme deviations from the mean that it becomes bad.'[6]

To determine averages, he needed a decent sample size – and an army provided the perfect testing ground. The Belgian statistician took published data listing the chest measurements of 5,738 Scottish soldiers. The differing chest sizes of these soldiers, Quetelet claimed, followed the same curve on a graph as 5,738 slightly mistaken measurements of the same man would.* By analogy, then, these real Scottish soldiers became *mistakes* on the error curve. They didn't just diverge from the average, they were imperfect copies of the ideal man, 'as though the chests which have been measured had been modelled from the same type from the same individual'.[7] The error curve had become a law of nature, not just a statistical measure of probability. Any movement away from the normal was basically a mistake, a deviation from the perfect human form designed by the creator. (For, unlike many later advocates of the normal, Quetelet was not an atheist.)

Quetelet's aesthetic ideals and social research crossed over in his interest in art and sculpture. He referred to his Scottish soldiers as 'living statues', their varied measurements a thousand slightly misshapen copies of the ancient Borghese Gladiator, a sculpture from *c*.100 BCE.[8] In his scientific treatises, too, the statistician outlined the study of the human body in artistic terms, from Ancient Greek sculpture to the Renaissance. His interest in physical form was inspired by Renaissance artists Leonardo da Vinci and Michelangelo, and by German artist and printmaker Albrecht Dürer's treatise on human proportions.[9] The notes in Quetelet's archive include studies comparing Egyptian mummies and nineteenth-century Belgians to the Medici Venus.

Yet, whereas Renaissance artists were often looking for variety as much as perfection (Leonardo da Vinci's inventory of his drawings early in his career included 'many

* Quetelet was not very painstaking with his data, and apparently made a number of mistakes copying from the original source. For more on this subject, see Stahl, 'The Evolution of the Normal Distribution', *Mathematics Magazine* 79, no. 2 (2006): 108–10.

necks of old women; many heads of old men'),[10] in Quetelet's time a scientific obsession with perfection and artistic ideals converged in the search for the average. This idea meant that ancient ideals embodied in crumbling statues infiltrated ordinary life as well as statistical knowledge. Contemporary tailors used the Apollo Belvedere – a Roman statue, now occasionally visible through the crowds in the Vatican Museum – as a stock model to construct their patterns.[11] Real bodies rarely measured up.

Although Quetelet had claimed the average man was a reflection of nature, later Europeans began to worry about the gap between what they saw around them and the classical ideal in height, body shape and appearance. The normal, they declared with horror, was no longer the average of a population (assuming that it ever had been) but that which *ought* to exist and rarely did. While Quetelet had proposed that the ideal body of the 'average man' was accompanied by a perfect moral mind, these later writers read immorality, idiocy and disease on to unusual bodies.

By plotting human characteristics on to an error curve, Quetelet did not just bring the study of statistical averages to social phenomena. He also set in place the belief that any deviation from the centre of the bell curve was some kind of aberration. His 'average man' was the first 'normal' human. The average man was, however, something of a paradox. He was at one and the same time a reflection of natural reality *and* an ideal for humanity to strive towards, flawless in body and in mind and the perfect representation of health.

A CENSUS OF HEALTH

What's the opposite of normal? Well, it depends on the context. If by normal we mean average, the opposite might be extreme or exceptional. Where normal means common its antonym could be unusual or strange. In medical terms, however, the opposite of normal has come to be pathological. If normal means healthy, the abnormal must be diseased.

This pairing only really entered medicine in the 1820s and became a common way of understanding health and illness for doctors. According to historians Peter Cryle and Elizabeth Stephens, it wasn't until well into the twentieth century that 'normal' became common in everyday speech, by which time the notion of normal as a statistical average and normal as an ideal state of health had merged.[12] The normal/pathological binary has shaped attitudes towards bodies and minds, towards sex and childhood development, ever since.

This is perhaps the area where the question of what's normal becomes most troubling for us today. If we are not normal, we wonder, does that mean we're sick? Concerns about the health and illness of populations were also one of the main reasons for the sharp increase in statistical collecting in the early 1800s. This obsession with numbers first became widespread during the great cholera epidemic that devastated Europe a few short years before Adolphe Quetelet unleashed the 'average man' on the world.

On 15 September 1832, cholera reached the Scottish market town of Dumfries, about twenty-five miles from the border with England. The bacterial disease, spread through contaminated water, causes severe and often fatal diarrhoea. At first, the pestilence seemed to be 'dallying with its work', with just one death a day. It was 'a heavy mortality in a population of ten thousand, yet not very alarming', remarked William McDowall, editor of the local newspaper, in his history of Dumfries published thirty-five years later.[13] By comparing the death rate to what was 'usual' in the population for the first time, the actual deaths in the cholera epidemic were understood differently from earlier epidemics.

Born in 1815, McDowall would have been a teenager during the outbreak, and remembered the subsequent panic well, describing it evocatively in his book. On 25 September, he tells us, fourteen cases and nine deaths were announced and 'all the people felt that the veritable plague was in their midst, and were filled with fear and trembling'. The doors of the high school were closed, hearses were seen in every street, and churches were vacated as people feared catching the disease from graves. By 3 October 'death was mercilessly titheing the town', which lay under a 'vast funeral pall' of cloud. By the end of the outbreak, 837 people had been diagnosed with cholera, and over half (421) had died. From the number of coffins made, however, McDowall suggests that the death toll was closer to 550: more than 5 per cent of the town's inhabitants.

The experience in Dumfries was not unusual in the severity of the outbreak. What *was* new was the numerical record of it. Across Europe, deaths from the cholera epidemic were widely reported, part of what philosopher Ian Hacking has called the 'avalanche of printed numbers' that characterised the decades 1820–1840.[14] From the census to records of crime, education, madness and disease, statistical information became widely used and understood in this period.

Not that this was the first time death rates had ever been recorded. In the early 1600s, weekly publication of the London Bills of Mortality warned civilians of the number of deaths from different causes across the city (including everything from 'Collick', to 'Winde' and 'Worms'), marking outbreaks of bubonic plague. In the nineteenth century, however, statistical collecting began to occur on a totally new scale across Europe. The first national census in both Britain and France was carried out in 1801. In France and Belgium, a tradition of numerical social studies was established by the 1820s. In Britain, a national statistics office was set up in 1832.[15] Changes in death or birth rates could now be set against what was 'normal' for the population in question.

The huge bureaucratic machines that enabled the collection of this data were at the heart of the emergence of the normal. The 'average man' was based on statistical analysis *and* huge amounts of population data. While the varying ways that statistics are recorded across nations continues to spark debate – as happened in the early stages of the Covid-19 pandemic in 2020 – the idea that numbers themselves are important is now widely accepted. This was simply not the case before the nineteenth century.

And of course, in such an age of statistics, Quetelet was not the only one to see a significance in the average or usual. In France, the physician François-Joseph-Victor Broussais drew large crowds to his Parisian lectures in the 1820s, where he described the differences between normal health and disease. There were no individual infections, the flamboyant revolutionary and liberal told his audience; *all* disease was caused by too much or too little irritation of the tissues.[16] As the philosopher Auguste Comte later put it, 'Until Broussais, the pathological state obeyed laws completely different from those governing the normal state, so that the exploration of the one could have no effect on the other.'[17] After Broussais, normal and pathological health were more often viewed on a continuum: different in degree, rather than in kind. This idea, rather helpfully, would soon come to be represented by the bell curve.

While these grand claims for a new system of medicine sounded ultra-modern to listeners at the time – and not a little controversial – the suggested method of treatment was a familiar and ancient one. The French doctor acquired the nickname 'the vampire of medicine' because of his great faith in the power of bloodletting. By the 1820s, leeching was all the rage in France, and even appeared in fashion: dresses with embroidered leeches became known as *les robes à la Broussais*.[18] Today we might dismiss Dr Broussais as a quack, but he genuinely believed in the therapeutic power of these bloodsucking creatures. He bled himself regularly for a variety of ailments, prescribing fifty or sixty at a time to cure his indigestion.

Although leeching made Broussais famous – and the subject of multiple cartoons – his new system of medicine was not as widely known. Outside the French-speaking world, the doctor's politics made his science seem suspicious by association: his leeching was spoken of as a bloody hangover from revolutionary France.[19] While a number of French and Belgian scientists began to adopt Broussais's

20

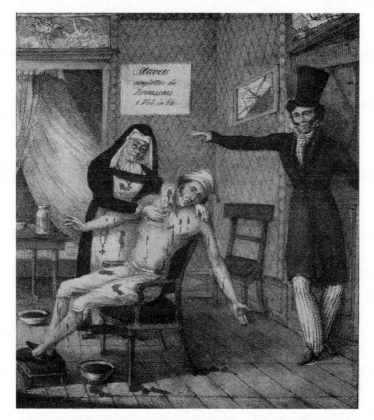

Caricature of Broussais demanding a nurse apply another fifty leeches to the patient, who protests that he has not a drop of blood left (undated, probably after 1832).

concept of the normal state of health, the doctor's influence was at first confined to these countries. It was not until Auguste Comte got involved that the idea spread across Europe.

Auguste Comte was Quetelet's contemporary. He was born just two years after the Belgian statistician, on 19 January 1798, in Montpellier near the south coast of France.

Revolutionary politics had a huge impact on Comte too. One of the main problems Comte dealt with in his philosophy was how to reorganise society in the post-revolutionary era. He even introduced a new secular form of religion: positivism.[20]

Comte claimed a universal significance for Broussais's medical system, just as Quetelet had done with the astronomer's error curve. In 1828 the philosopher picked up Broussais's newly published *On Irritation and Madness* and declared his support for the idea that disease states arose from deviations in intensity of the same principles that governed normal health. This idea was not only applicable to internal disease states; according to Comte, it applied to *everything*.

There were personal reasons for Comte's interest in this particular treatise; he had recently recovered from a psychotic episode. On 12 April 1826, Comte's friends and colleagues – including, according to Comte's biographer, Broussais himself – waited outside the philosopher's apartments for the fourth lecture in a year-long series.[21] The blinds were down, the door closed, and the crowd eventually dispersed, assuming that their lecturer was ill. Over the next week, several friends received rather rambling notes from the philosopher. Eventually Comte's wife, Caroline – a former washerwoman the young man had married the previous February – found her husband in the suburb of Montmorency, his favourite part of Paris. He was in the process of setting fire to his hotel room and Caroline decided her husband was insane. On 18 April, Comte was diagnosed with mania and admitted to a private asylum.

Here, the young philosopher was sedated and kept isolated. He was emotionally excitable and, to calm him, he was prescribed baths, cold showers and, yes, the application of leeches. Despite these most modern of remedies, on 2 December Comte was discharged as incurable. On the journey home, he told his wife and friends that the Austerlitz Bridge was the Golden Horn in Istanbul. When one of the party corrected the philosopher, Comte punched him. At home, Auguste was uncommunicative and isolated, beset by fantasies. During a dinner-time argument with his wife and mother, the philosopher tried to cut his throat with a table knife. Caroline decided on an unusual approach for the time: she would remove any signs of madness from their home. She dismissed the attendant Auguste's psychiatrist had sent and removed the bars from the windows. She took the same medicines, so that her husband would not think she treated him differently. Immediately, she claimed, the philosopher began to improve and, in six weeks, Caroline thought him completely recovered.

If only it had been so easy. In reality it seems to have taken closer to two years, with a spell of deep depression and a further suicide attempt in early 1827.[22] It was about this time that Comte wrote his paper on Broussais's treatise, remarking on the insight he had gained through 'personal experience'.[23] It was this experience that led him to support the thesis that normal and abnormal were different in degree rather than in kind.

What did this shift in thinking mean? Well, for Comte it was not just health that could be normal or pathological. Any human action, custom, practice, belief or notion could also fit on the same scale. While people before this time certainly mocked or shunned the behaviour of neighbours who did not meet a standard expected by the community, the idea that aberrant actions could be equated with disease gave a new urgency to this need to conform. It also implied – even if this was not Comte's intention – that the social codes that informed these decisions were fixed and unchanging.

Social expectations change all the time. You might have seen the memes popular on social media listing the reasons for admission to Victorian asylums, from over-study to disappointment in love. While presented rather misleadingly – these were suggested by doctors to be the root cause of an unusual state of mind such as melancholy, delusions or mania, not evidence of illness itself – they certainly do show how unusual behaviour is invariably interpreted through the social codes of an era. Study – and especially reading medical or antiquarian texts – was thought especially dangerous behaviour for women, something that never failed to amuse me as a woman studying the history of medicine. When Edith Cotton refused to wear a hat out of doors in 1898, this was deemed a sign of mental illness, because wearing a hat was right and proper.[24] Meanwhile, after her mother died in 1881, young Amy Dorrell began 'constantly going to church' and 'always reading the Bible', behaviour that might have seemed normal in earlier centuries or other communities where religious observance was a more constant presence in people's lives.[25] While late Victorian doctors certainly debated the line between eccentricity and madness, thanks to Broussais and Comte they did not doubt for a moment that the two states were linked; gradations on a curve of health.[26]

But it wasn't just individuals who were singled out on this spectrum of eccentricity and madness, health and disease. Around the same time, a more sinister chapter in the history of the normal began, as the idea of who was normal – and what behaviours and beliefs were acceptable – expanded to take in whole groups and communities. Because the story of the normal is also a story of exclusion, it has often operated along lines of class, race, gender and religious belief as scientists aimed 'to confirm or perfect sociological laws' to first understand, and then control, the moral and intellectual functions of humankind.[27]

THE LIMITS OF THE NORMAL

On 20 December 1899, writer William Corner was pleased to see an advert in *The Times* calling for volunteers to fight in South Africa. Despite his age being 'more years than I care to tell beyond that limit which the War Office decided was admissible or compatible with efficiency', Corner immediately went to sign up.[28] After a few minor bureaucratic hurdles – including the closure of one office because the furniture had not arrived – he eventually gained an interview. This was followed by a medical examination and rifle and riding tests. 'A few good men fell by the wayside,' Corner – or Private No. 6243, as he became – remarked in his history of the 34th Company (Middlesex) Imperial Yeomanry. This 'was a pity, for neither doctors, range sergeants, nor riding-masters are infallible, and there are so many compensating qualifications as to fitness or unfitness in the field of active service'. It was, he concluded, 'made so difficult for a willing man to serve his country'.[29]

William Corner's medical examination no doubt included measurement of his height and chest size. During conflict, the usual military requirements were often reduced because more recruits were needed – as had presumably happened in the case of Corner's age. In 1861, prospective soldiers were expected to be at least 5 foot 8, but by 1900 this had been reduced to 5 foot 3.[30] Even so, not everyone, as Corner noted, met these criteria.

For some commentators, this became proof that industrial city life had caused a decline in working men's bodies. In Manchester, reported polemicist Arnold White, 11,000 men tried to sign up for the Boer War between October 1899 and July 1900. A full 8,000 were rejected outright and, of the 3,000 accepted, less than half 'attained the moderate standard of muscular power and chest measurement required by the military authorities'.[31] Examples like this betrayed the 'characteristic *physical* type of town dweller: stunted, narrow-chested, easily wearied'.[32]

White's figures – for which he gave no source – have since been questioned and were not even accepted by all readers at the time. He was a known troublemaker in political circles, and his *Efficiency and Empire* goes on to outline his antisemitic and eugenic views in unpleasant detail.[33] Nonetheless, concern over Britain's male bodies in the Boer War campaign did lead to questions in Parliament and the appointment of a government inquiry. The threat of physical degeneration, particularly of the poor, fuelled a moral panic that had begun several decades earlier, showing how the changing size and shape of bodies has, since the mid-nineteenth century, been used to illustrate or justify wider fears about society.

The fear of degeneration spread across Europe around the turn of the twentieth century as scientists began to worry about the 'failure of natural selection in the case of man', as writer William Rathbone Greg called it.[34] Since, as Charles Darwin claimed, man had the 'great power of adapting his habits to new conditions of life' – building shelter, making clothes, or inventing tools and weapons – Greg argued that natural selection had been unable to operate on human biology in the same way it did in other species.[35] When animals get sick or injured, he said, they die – but humans have doctors and hospitals. If animals cannot find food, they die – yet humans support each other. Darwin concluded that this proved the moral superiority of humankind and aided the mental evolution of the species; other scientists were divided. What most of them agreed on, however, was that civilisation itself was changing the physical and mental norms of humanity.

From French doctor Bénédict Morel's treatise on the hereditary transmission of physical, intellectual and moral traits (1857) to Hungarian-born physician and journalist Max Nordau's attack on the intellectual and artistic world (1892), degeneration became the buzzword of the fin de siècle. This discussion was most often applied to the physical decline of the working man – as in the Boer War controversy – and popularly associated with modernity and city life. While height and weight were often interpreted as signs of degeneration, so too were countless other physical signs. In *Degeneration of Londoners* (1885) Scottish surgeon James Cantlie described how Londoners were made pale, emaciated, stunted and miserable by their smoggy, overcrowded living conditions. In this dark, polluted atmosphere, one twenty-one-year-old man had grown to just 5 foot 1, with a chest measurement of 28 inches, a full 12 inches below the ideal Scottish soldier-cum-Borghese Gladiator described by Quetelet. The lad's head was small, his aspect 'pale waxy'. The gap between his eyes was narrow, he had a decided squint and he was intensely solemn. (If Cantlie took an 8 a.m. Tube journey today he would doubtless be horrified by the degenerate solemnity of the waxy faces all around him.)

Degenerating bodies permeated Victorian fiction. In Robert Louis Stevenson's well-known story of a respected professional entering into a drug-induced primitive state, *Strange Case of Dr Jekyll and Mr Hyde* (1886), Hyde differs physically as well as mentally from Dr Jekyll. Hyde is 'pale and dwarfish' – like Cantlie's young Londoners – and 'gave an impression of deformity without any nameable malformation'.[36] While Mr Hyde makes his appearance as a result of Jekyll's mistaken faith in the inevitability of scientific progress, he is also a product of the city. Dr Jekyll lives in the medical heartland of London, on spacious Cavendish Square in Westminster: a street coloured the wealthiest yellow on Charles Booth's 1889 London poverty map.[37] The doctor takes rooms for Hyde, however, in nearby Soho, the seedy underbelly of the West End. Vice, the city and physical decline went hand in hand in the Victorian popular mind as London became the 'city of dreadful delight', in the words of historian Judith Walkowitz.[38]

The science of degeneration collided with the science of the normal in the work of Victorian polymath Francis

Galton. Galton – Charles Darwin's younger cousin – was one of the first scientists to call the error curve the 'normal distribution' (in 1877), among his many other contributions to science.[39] He developed and popularised influential theories in statistics, founded psychometric testing, and contributed to the development of fingerprinting. He also coined the term eugenics. Galton's self-professed 'race science' would improve the national stock by encouraging the 'fit' (him and his wealthy friends) to have more children and the 'unfit' (the working classes, people of colour, and anyone who didn't meet an arbitrary physical or mental standard) to have fewer, perhaps even preventing certain people from breeding at all. This was hardly a fringe project: eugenics infiltrated much of Western science and medicine in the late nineteenth and early twentieth centuries. And, until at least 1950 – when the name was finally changed – the well-respected University College London (UCL) housed the Galton Laboratory for National Eugenics.*

The two things can't be separated from each other. Galton's interests in statistics, normality, identity and heredity were bound up in his concerns with and promotion of eugenics. This point is often missed. When the Museum of London put on a (mostly quite good) Sherlock Holmes exhibition in 2014, the final room included a range of scientific equipment from the Galton collection. 'Francis Galton was a scientist in London at the same time Sherlock Holmes

* In 2018, UCL launched an inquiry into the history of eugenics at the university, following revelations in the press that secret conferences on eugenics and intelligence had been held at UCL since 2015. The inquiry resulted in the renaming of the Galton Lecture Theatre (as well as rooms associated with Galton's protégé, Karl Pearson), and sadly very little else. Anna Fazackerley, 'UCL Eugenics Inquiry Did Not Go Far Enough, Committee Say', *Guardian*, 28 February 2020.

was solving crimes in the city,' announced the display label (I'm paraphrasing, of course). 'Here's some equipment a bit like what Sherlock Holmes might have used.' Most exhibition visitors had probably never heard of Galton. 'What a genius!' they might have gone away thinking, if they remembered him at all. They would not have considered the way his fingerprinting techniques were used to advance colonial rule, or the devastating effects eugenics had around the world on people deemed to be 'other'.

Galton was interested in variation, not just averages.[40] He distributed sweet pea seeds among his friends, sorted by the size of their parent plants, in an effort to measure the effect of inheritance on height. He set up a pop-up Anthropometric Laboratory at the International Health Exhibition of 1884, where members of the public could pay a small fee to measure their height, grip strength, visual acuity and countless other characteristics – handily giving himself data on thousands of visitors. And he applied the normal distribution to countless human traits and characteristics, a far wider range than even Quetelet had done.[41] Indeed, Galton was so positive that heredity and genius were intimately related that he claimed that a normal distribution of 'talents' from his own research showed exactly the same thing as a distribution of social class using the figures of industrialist and social reformer Charles Booth. If class and talent were the same, he said (a staggeringly ridiculous claim), then the class structure of Victorian society was both natural and, you guessed it, normal. Galton's disciple, Karl Pearson, despite professing socialist and feminist beliefs in his youth, agreed that 'very poor persons who subsist on casual earnings' were also those with the least talents and 'from the standpoint of civic worth ... are undesirables'.[42] Once again, normal standards could lead to a casually dismissive determination of who was – and was not – worthwhile as a human being, based purely on circumstantial evidence.

Not all Galton's work on the normal was statistical. I've long found his 'composite' photographs particularly fascinating. In 1878, with the help of evolutionary psychologist Herbert Spencer, Galton reported that he had found a way of 'extracting the typical characteristics' from a group of persons 'alike in most respects'.[43] This method relied on the long photographic exposure times of the 1870s. Galton would take eight portraits of the same size and arrange them pinned one in front of the other so that the eyes were roughly in line. If the exposure time for an exact copy of an image was eighty seconds, Galton would remove a picture every ten seconds so that each photograph was only briefly exposed. When the plate was developed it would show a picture that 'represents no man in particular, but portrays an imaginary figure, possessing the average features of any given group of men'.[44] The average man had become visible.

Galton's early portraits were of violent criminals, and he expected the composites to highlight their 'criminal features'. These were described by his contemporary, Italian criminologist Cesare Lombroso, to include cheek-pouches, a flattened nose and angular skull and excessively sized eye sockets 'which, combined with the hooked nose, so often imparts to criminals the aspects of birds of prey'.[45] To Galton's surprise, instead of highlighting these attributes, the composites served to soften them. The 'special villainous

SPECIMENS OF COMPOSITE PORTRAITURE

PERSONAL AND FAMILY.

 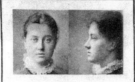

Alexander the Great From 6 Different Medals.

Two Sisters.

From 6 Members of same Family Male & Female.

HEALTH.	DISEASE.	CRIMINALITY,

6 Cases

8 Cases

9 Cases

4 Cases

23 Cases. Royal Engineers, 12 Officers, 11 Privates

Tubercular Disease

2 Of the many Criminal Types

CONSUMPTION AND OTHER MALADIES

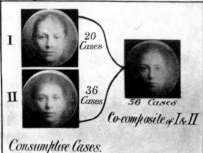 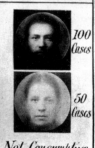

I   *20 Cases*

100 Cases

II   *36 Cases*

56 Cases Co-composite of I & II

50 Cases

Consumptive Cases.

Not Consumptive.

A selection of composite photographs published by Galton in 1883, aiming to show typical diseases as well as criminals. Consumption (tuberculosis) was widely presumed to be hereditary at the time.

irregularities' of the criminals faded so that 'the common humanity that underlies them has prevailed'. While this could have been taken to mean that there was no such thing as a typical criminal, Galton was not so ready to let go of hereditary biology. The composite photograph represented for Galton, 'not the criminal, but the man who is liable to fall into crime'; it was not the average of every man, but only of certain abnormal men.[46] Galton believed that his photographs supported the idea that there was such a thing as 'average' criminal features, and that someone pre-disposed to crime could be physically identified. So could many other 'types' of person, from the mentally ill to tuber-culosis patients. The abnormal character or mind of these groups would appear on the composite face.

But what *was* normal for Francis Galton and his followers? It's crucial to remember that Galton already had quite a specific idea of normal before he began to represent the notion on a bell curve, as a study by Peter Cryle and Elizabeth Stephens has shown.[47] This is a trend that we see time and time again. Galton and his fellow scientists removed data that was thought to be irregular from their figures before they even calculated their norms. Children – with their infuriating tendency to grow as they progress in years – had long been a problem for statisticians. But so too were women. Galton 'transmuted' the female data he gathered to make it directly comparable to men – women's heights, for example, had to be increased using an equation he devised so that the data would continue to fit a bell curve.

This adaptation was not only a statistical device for comparison. It also resulted in setting a standard: men were the biological normal to which female data had to be adapted. And, of course, white men were the norm to which other races were to be compared. In the late Victorian era, the middle-class white professional became the new average man. He – for the normal standard remained exclusively male – was a doctor, scientist, writer, banker, merchant, lawyer or businessman. He was not the most common type of person, statistically speaking, but he was nonetheless held to be the healthy ideal by which others should be judged. It was he who could afford the time and expense to take up James Cantlie's prescription of cycling and lawn tennis to keep the spectre of the city's Mr Hyde at bay. He might also join the Alpine Club, as psychiatrist George Savage did, to be approvingly described by his friends as a 'vigorous climber' who 'revelled in climbing crags, sport on the moors … and skiing over snow and icy roads'.[48]

Conversely, the 'failure' of those in certain social classes and ethnic groups to reach the ideal height, weight or chest circumference of the middle-class professional was widely understood as a social problem. Stunted growth was not caused by environment and circumstance, many Victorians assumed, but biological inheritance and moral failing. Therefore, according to eugenic theory, certain people had to be prevented from having children. While marriage licences were never introduced in Britain – although plenty of doctors, scientists, politicians and other commentators advocated for them – in the US and Europe legal statutes enforcing marriage restrictions and sterilisations emerged in the first few decades of the twentieth century. The world's first compulsory sterilisation law was passed in Indiana in 1907, intended to prevent those deemed physically and mentally 'unfit' from having children of their own.[49]

This obsession with physical decline was inextricable from discrimination and anxieties around race, as well as class. Scientists compared 'degenerate' white English-men to so-called primitive races. They ranked races and classes based on skull size and shape, as well as height, weight and physical characteristics.[50] Victorian writers christened Africa the 'dark continent' and found its twin in the East End of London.[51] 'This summer the attention of the civilised world has been arrested by the story which Mr Stanley has told of "Darkest Africa",' wrote William Booth, founder of the Salvation Army, in language that shocks today but was accepted unthinkingly by most of Booth's white readership at the time. Booth spoke of the 'wooded wilderness' of the Congo Basin where 'in the dark, dank air, filled with the steam of the heated morass, human beings dwarfed into pygmies and brutalised into cannibals lurk and live and die'.[52] Booth took this pejorative description by explorer Henry Stanley for granted and concluded: 'As there is a darkest Africa is there not also a darkest England?'[53] For Booth and other missionaries, religion was the 'way out' of such 'uncivilised' circumstances. For Stanley – more famous today for uttering the words 'Dr Livingstone, I presume?' than his role in the Belgian colonisation of central Africa – international trade was the civilising force. For Galton and his colleagues, of course, science was the essential tool of normalisation.

While Galton's eugenic theories have thankfully been discredited – though rather more recently than you might expect – the prescriptive and hierarchical notion of a white, masculine, cisgendered normal remains in place across much of science and medicine, and in the charts and measurements we still use today. It has supported negative attitudes and stereotypes that we can still easily find across the internet and in our social media feeds. And some of the standards we accept unthinkingly are built on deeply skewed nineteenth- and early twentieth-century studies. Figures for healthy weight and blood pressure, for example, originated in the first half of the twentieth century from statistics gathered by US insurance companies, whose policies were primarily purchased by better-off white Americans. It is only very recently that it has been recognised that the link between BMI and health varies for different body types: people of Asian descent may have a higher risk of diabetes and heart disease at a size that would be deemed 'normal' for white Europeans, while Black women have a lower risk of health problems at larger sizes.[54]

The Galton collection today is packed away in a rather unremarkable storage cabinet, similar to the sort you might keep office stationery in. The bulk of Galton's papers and photographs are in the UCL library's special collections; this cupboard contains the oddments that don't fit into an archive – the contents of Galton's desk at the time of his death, equipment attached to his major discoveries and a random assortment of personal effects.

Other, more sinister items were added later, speaking to the devastating legacy of eugenics. A long metal tin is labelled simply 'Haarfarbenfafel von Prof Dr Eugen Fischer'. Inside are thirty different bunches of synthetic hair, each neatly labelled with a number: Fischer's hair colour gauge. German scientist Fischer used this gauge in Namibia in 1908 to judge the relative 'whiteness' of mixed-race people under colonial rule. His study took a fiercely eugenic approach. He recommended the prevention of mixed marriage and supported the genocide of Herero and Nama people in what was then German Southwest Africa. In 1912, interracial marriage was prohibited throughout German colonies, following Fischer's recommendations. Adolf Hitler was inspired to write *Mein Kampf* in part by Fischer's promotion of eugenics, and his work became scientific support for the antisemitic Nuremberg laws that led to the Holocaust. The scientist officially joined the Nazi Party in 1940.[55]

Since Fischer was using the hair gauge in 1908, just a few years before Galton's death, it is likely that it was sent to Karl Pearson rather than Galton himself.* Yet the gauge does show the extent to which eugenics was taken in the twentieth century. When the *Guardian* newspaper announced in 2018 that UCL was holding an inquiry into eugenics, it reported the objections of one lecturer that linking Galton 'with the Nazis is an horrific sentimentalist slur'.[56] Yet the collection itself shows a direct link from Galton's protégé to a Nazi scientist: significantly fewer than six degrees of separation.

The Laboratory for National Eugenics at UCL remained in existence after the Second World War. So too did eugenic sterilisation programmes in parts of Europe and North America, which aimed to prevent certain groups judged 'abnormal' from having children. In the Czech

---

* Pearson and Fischer certainly corresponded. In 1932, Fischer wrote to Pearson to congratulate him on having been awarded the Rudolf Virchow medal, and asking if one of Fischer's colleagues could come to England to give a talk to the Eugenics Education Society. Letter from Fischer to Pearson, October 1932, UCL Special Collections (PEARSON/11/1/6/21).

Republic, to take just one example, forced sterilisation of Romani women *began* in 1971, with the last known case as recent as 2007.[57]

Victorian polymath Francis Galton and Nazi scientist Eugen Fischer may have been very different people, working in very different environments. But their stories, and their legacies, show just how dangerous the concept of 'normal' can be, and the power that it holds. Both Galton and Fischer used their interests in classifying bodies and minds to decide who was normal, to marginalise – and worse – those who did not fit these criteria, and, most sinisterly, to suggest how humanity might be intentionally altered to fit a white, elite ideal: a chilling chapter in the history of the so-called normal.

AM I NORMAL?

When I left school in 1997, I was filled with immense relief. I was escaping the small-town bullies and dull conformists of my youth. I was moving to London for university, a magical city where, it seemed to me, people could do as they liked and no one blinked an eye. As an awestruck teenager, I marvelled at the diversity around me. As a white heterosexual woman I was also undoubtedly blind to much of the racism, homophobia, ableism and transphobia around me. At times, I no doubt unwittingly contributed to it. I had no understanding of the legacy of colonialism or eugenics, or the way racist norms continued to shape the structure of society. My notion of normality was individual, naïve and self-centred. I even refused to call myself a feminist.

London, I thought then, was a place where you could be what and who you liked; a city teeming with variety yet cloaked in comforting anonymity. There was something for everyone, and a safety in the ever-moving crowd. I still love London, and it still feels like home in a way the Kentish town I grew up in never did. But I had a rude awakening from my romantic expectations when I moved into a tower block in South Woodford – 'practically *Essex*!' my fellow students and I bitterly agreed. I shared a floor with twelve other eighteen- and nineteen-year-old girls. For some reason I had thought they'd be more accepting than my peers at school. They weren't. They gossiped and giggled and made snide remarks – sometimes in person, sometimes behind the battered old doors and thin walls of the student halls. Even those who weren't part of the clique would pause mid-conversation and stare accusingly at me. 'You're so *quiet*!' was their constant refrain. It felt like a cruel reprimand; a sign that I was not like them. I never quite dared to answer as I really wanted: 'So what?'

The stupid thing was that I knew some of those girls who wore a lot of make-up and loved superficial gossip worried about fitting in just as I did. After giggling and bitching with her friends, my next-door neighbour would cry to her boyfriend late at night. 'I hate it here!' I'd hear her wail through the wall. After just one term, she dropped out. By the end of the year, I discovered that a surprising number of other people disliked this group that I had thought of as the popular one. Maybe they weren't the ideal after all?

Yet knowing both these things did not change my fears. The idea of being normal was so deep-rooted that it survived the knowledge that my persecutors had the same worries as me, and that those I thought of as 'normal' were not particularly well liked. I retained the desire to 'correct' myself even as I gained the strength to reject them.

Our ideas of normality fall somewhere between our desire for individuality and our need to be accepted as part of a group. Fitting in can have value, even if it might not always be possible, and may sometimes be damaging to our mental and physical health. But if the emerging awareness that the norms we grow up with are not as universal as we once believed cannot shake our faith in the normal itself, perhaps its history can.

It would certainly have surprised me, as a shy eighteen-year-old, to learn that people had not always divided the world into normal and abnormal. A seventeenth-century Cornish fisherman might have compared himself to other local fishermen, to his family or to his neighbours, but he most certainly didn't worry about where he fitted in some overarching scheme of normality. To learn that, two short centuries ago, people didn't even use the word normal to describe human attributes or experiences at all, reduces the power of the concept at least a little.

Over the years, as I read more about the history of medicine and science, about colonialism and gender, about queer theory and the social model of disability, my notion of the normal gradually became a little less self-indulgent, a little less insular. I realised that, despite my experiences and anxiety, I was privileged. By luck of birth, I had grown up closer to the Western so-called norm than many people, even if I had felt far from normal at a selective state school in a wealthy part of southern England.

The normal is both personal and political. A critique of being normal can best begin with an awareness of our place within it, a careful interrogation of the expectations and assumptions we grew up with and the ways these are embedded in our institutions, our laws, our politics and our social interactions. That's what I try to do in this book.

But who ultimately gets to decide what's normal anyway? Quetelet, Broussais, Comte, Galton, Pearson and their fellow scientists would all have claimed that no such decision occurred. They thought they were recording – objectively and dispassionately – something that merely existed, whether that thing was God's masterplan or a law of nature or evolutionary science. The way their statistics were collected, however, and the frameworks they used to analyse them, all relied on human interpretation. They included certain criteria and discarded others to create their so-called scientific norms, based on white, well-off, Western men.

Although the ideas and methodologies of these nine-teenth-century scientists essentialised the normal as a yardstick for human lives and behaviours, in actual fact there *was* no clear answer as to what constituted a normal body, normal health or a normal type of person. The determination of all of these things relied on social expectations and attitudes, which have altered drastically through time and across cultures. The way these norms have changed, as the rest of this book will show, leads us back time and again to this question: is there really any such thing as normal?

2

DO I HAVE A
NORMAL BODY?

I have always loathed buying shoes.

That's not just because it's difficult to find anything to fit my oversized feet – hard though that undoubtedly is. It's also the invariable reaction of the salesperson, which ranges from horrified incredulity to disbelief. As a teenager, I would shrivel up inside every time someone greeted my whispered 'Do you have this in a 9?' with an astounded shriek of 'Size 9?!' Yes, I have big feet: a 9 in England, 43 if you're European, 11 if you're in the US. As a result, I spent most of my youth wearing the same pair of unisex trainers or DMs until they fell apart.

I still hate buying shoes.

What's surprised me, though, over the twenty-five or so years that I've had this problem is the number of other women I've met with size 9 or 10 feet. And yet the sizes available in stores haven't really changed in all that time. A handful of cheap high-street shops do a 9 in the occasional shoe but, in the UK, most women's ranges still stop at size

8. Yet our feet are apparently getting bigger. A 2014 survey by the College of Podiatry suggested that feet in the UK have gone up by two shoe sizes since the 1970s: the average size for a man has risen from 8 to 10, and for a woman from 4 to 6.[1] This would suggest larger shoe sizes are more common than they were fifty years ago. If we assume the distribution for foot size in the UK matches that in the US, it would make 'normal' size for women (95 per cent of the population) between a size 3 and a 9.[2] So 9 is normal after all.

The example of the humble shoe illustrates several things. The first is that the normal body is shaped not just by what's usual, but also by a range of cultural factors and expectations (including what shoe shops decide to sell). Both senses of normal affect our ideas of the size a foot should be, but cultural expectations are especially influential. After all, if it had been easy for teenage me to buy shoes and no one had batted an eyelid when I asked for my size, I would probably never have thought of my feet as unusually huge. The history of consumer choice, then, has a large part to play in our ideas about normal bodies. When it was common for people to make their own clothes, comparing your size with that of other people was less significant.

The second thing is the way concerns about the changing size and shape of our bodies have been used to illustrate or justify wider fears about human populations. A BBC article about the shoe size survey cited above jumped from discussing larger feet to the so-called 'obesity epidemic'. 'Feet are getting bigger because as a nation we are becoming taller and we're increasing in weight,' Lorraine Jones from the College of Podiatry was quoted as saying, which the BBC interpreted to mean that 'our feet have compensated by growing longer and wider'. Yet it is not clear that the survey measured height or weight as well as shoe size and no definite evidence is given for the connection. Large feet are nonetheless represented by the media as a sign of decline in physical health – rather missing the point of the CoP study, which was primarily concerned about people damaging their feet by wearing shoes that don't fit. This kind of link appears repeatedly through the history of the normal body. We have already seen how different parts of the body have been read as evidence of degeneration of the species or national decline, as well as justification for colonial expansion or in support of racist and sexist hierarchies of civilisation.

Finally, there's the role medicine has played in the relationship we have with our own bodies. At one and the same time we feel part of and distinct from our bodies. As the French philosopher Paul Valéry put it, we might speak of our body 'as of a thing that belongs to us; but for us it is not entirely a thing; and it belongs to us a little less than we belong to it'.[3] I first came across this quote in Shigehisa Kuriyama's fascinating history of the divergence of Greek and Chinese medicine, which shows how bodies have been interpreted and conceived of very differently in different medical traditions. In the first and second centuries CE, Greek doctors saw muscles where Chinese doctors saw a system of acupuncture tracts and points. Kuriyama tells us that Chinese didn't even have a specific word for 'muscle'.

This was not a case of one tradition seeing 'correctly'. Neither model was externally visible on most human bodies.

Indeed, it was common in medical practice at this time *not* to distinguish between different types of flesh. The Greeks were the odd ones out, their anatomy rooted in an artistic tradition depicting bulging, naked men, rippling even in places where muscles don't anatomically exist.[4] The very ways of viewing our own bodies, then, are just as bound up in history and culture as the judgements we make about whether or not what we see is normal.

BEAUTY MYTHS

In September 1945, the *Cleveland Plain Dealer* newspaper launched a competition under the headline 'Are you Norma, Typical Woman?' Entrants were asked to submit their measurements, from height and weight to bust, hip, waist, thigh, calf and foot size. The aim was to find the woman who best fitted a sculpture created by sexologist Robert L. Dickinson and sculptor Abram Belskie in 1942.[5] Normman and Norma – as the Dickinson-Belskie statues were known – captured both a statistical average and an ideal. Their bodies were formed from the measurements of thousands of American men and women, and they were thus supposed to represent normal Americans. Yet both were based on a heavily selected sample: young people, aged around eighteen to twenty, able-bodied, healthy and – revealingly – almost exclusively white. The pair were even labelled 'Native White American' when displayed to the public, further associating the normal American with whiteness, while simultaneously erasing from history the American peoples who pre-dated European colonisation.[6]

Nearly 4,000 women entered the competition, yet not a single one matched Norma's measurements precisely. Winner Martha Skidmore was simply the woman who came closest. Although presented as both an average *and* an all-American ideal, it turned out that Norma as a person was entirely fictional.[7] This revelation did not, unfortunately, overturn the ideals associated with normal female beauty.

Well before Norma, the demands associated with appearance weighed more heavily on women than on men. When asylum inspectors visited the Bethlem Royal Hospital in the nineteenth century, it was often the improperly dressed female patients they passed disapproving comment on. This did not mean that the male inhabitants were any less dishevelled. It was simply that men were not judged by their appearance to the same extent. For a woman in Britain at that time, wearing her hair down or going out

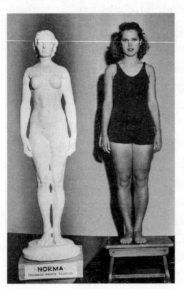

without a hat was thought to reveal more about her state of mind or character than similar behaviour said about a man.

I can't remember a time when I wasn't aware of this double standard. Growing up in the 1980s, I knew that the expectations placed on me as a girl did not affect my male friends in the same

Martha Skidmore, winner of the 1945 'Norma' look-a-like competition, photographed next to the statue of Norma, average woman.

way. Aged three, I dealt with this by insisting that I was not Sarah, I was a little boy called Mark. My favourite item of clothing – until my friend Paul stole it – was a purple tie. Before starting primary school, my best friend and I made a pact that we would never wear skirts or dresses other than the hated but obligatory school uniform. I was furious at the teacher who insisted she needed 'big strong boys' to help her move things in the classroom, given that we were six and there were just as many big strong girls in the class. And when, aged eight, I was told that, as a girl, it was no longer appropriate for me to play football at school my frustration turned inward. I increasingly wished I *was* a boy. As a teenager I would regularly turn the bedroom mirror to face the wall. I wore ever-increasing layers of shirts and baggy T-shirts to hide my hated body, but it was the tail-end of grunge, so no one really noticed. It wasn't until I was well into my twenties that I started to reflect on the complicated relationship between gender and appearance in my life. Maybe it wasn't my body that was abnormal after all. Perhaps it was the way the world treated women that was the problem. Or even the very idea of gender itself.

Since the 1990s, numerous studies have shown that body dissatisfaction among women has become 'normative' in the Western world.[8] Most women worry about their appearance, a concern lying somewhere between a norm ('am I the correct dress size?') and an ideal ('do I have perfect skin, hair or teeth?'). Of course, men also suffer concerns about their appearance, and many people have fears that lie outside this binary notion of gender. Expectations about appearance may be particularly challenging for women who were not born female, while attitudes to gender can be starkly visible to someone who identifies as non-binary. Appearance remains, however, something that is commonly – and often unpleasantly – associated with gender.

It was certainly women, and not men, who were the subjects of one of Francis Galton's 'beauty' experiments. In the Francis Galton collection at University College London, a pair of 'registrators' are discreetly tucked away in a basement drawer. When I mention Galton's 'creepy beauty gloves', the curator immediately knows which object I'm talking about. The smart leather gloves were modified by Galton to enable him to count in secret: the left glove has a pin in the thumb and a pad of felt across the four fingers. Galton placed a strip of paper over the felt and then, by touching different fingers with the pin, could keep track of what he saw without anyone's knowledge. 'Whenever you can, count' was Galton's motto, according to his protégé Karl Pearson; a bit like the Sesame Street vampire.[9]

The creepy gloves came in handy when Galton decided to grade the relative beauty of women across Great Britain. The eminent statistician stood on street corners in different cities, hands twitching dubiously inside his coat pockets every time a woman passed by. Galton graded the beauty of the women he saw, from attractive to indifferent to repellent. On the basis of this entirely subjective study, the scientist aimed to create a beauty map of Britain, though it was never completed.[10] Nonetheless, Galton did conclude that women in his native London were the most beautiful, while those in Aberdeen were the most repellent. Not that it's all that surprising that the hair, make-up and clothing of London ladies were more appealing to a fellow capital-dweller than the fashions of a windswept fishing port. However, it does seem a wonder dear Frank wasn't arrested.

While sleazy by modern standards, Galton was not personally to blame for the scientific objectification of women. He simply participated in a practice that was widespread. Male Victorian scientists tended to assume that women's natural place was in the home, giving birth to and raising children. The main function of a young woman, then, was to attract a husband, and therefore her beauty had evolutionary value. Darwin, in his theory of sexual selection, saw female beauty as instrumental in the marriages of mankind. He referred to the 'selection during many generations of those women, which appear to the men of each race the most attractive'.[11] Oddly, this was in direct contrast with what the evolutionary biologist described in the animal kingdom, where males were more colourful or decorated in order to attract a mate. While a peahen might have her choice of dazzling peacocks, in humans the opposite was apparently true.

Despite adapting his theories to fit social expectation, Darwin did acknowledge that there was no such thing as a universal standard of beauty. Yet, while he spent a long time describing the facial features and skin tones considered beautiful in other parts of the world, those deemed attractive by Europeans seemed so obvious as to require no description at all: the sole characteristic to gain a passing mention was women's long hair.[12] This was thanks to traveller and social Darwinist William Winwood Reade, who claimed that long hair in women was both universally admired *and* the result of sexual selection for 'by the continued selection of long-haired wives the flowing tresses of the sex have been produced'.[13] Perhaps Reade was unaware that it is entirely possible for men to grow their hair long or women to cut their 'flowing tresses' short; like Darwin he saw long hair as a biological characteristic and not a social norm. Men should remember that 'the elegance of the female form, its softness of complexion, its gracefulness of curve are not less our creation than the symmetry and speed of the racehorse, the magnificence of garden flowers, and the flavour of orchard fruits'.[14] Well done men for breeding such perfect women and racehorses.

Although these writers were extremely vague about what was beautiful in a woman, the examples they gave drew on racial hierarchies of difference, developed in the colonial period. Darwin, for example, assumed that flat noses were unattractive, an attitude cultural historian Sander Gilman dates to late eighteenth-century anthropological studies.[15] Petrus Camper, the eighteenth-century Dutch anatomist, developed a theory of beauty measured by the nasal index and facial angle. The first was a line drawn from the forehead, across the nose to the upper lip. This was intersected by the latter, a horizontal line from the jaw. The most beautiful face, according to Camper, was one in which the two lines lay at an angle of 100 degrees.[16]

Again, this was linked to classical art – Roman sculptures had an angle of 96 degrees, and Ancient Greek statues the perfect 100 degrees (though whether their models were actually quite so beautiful, Camper himself was sceptical). The eighteenth-century European was less beautiful, at around 80 degrees. Even so, this study claimed to lend scientific weight to the idea that white Europeans were the most beautiful race in the modern world; in other races the angle was even lower. So, while Darwin drew attention to different standards of beauty across cultures, he and most of his contemporaries nonetheless applied a hierarchy to facial features based on race. Large eyes, an oval face, high-bridged nose, narrow lips and a defined chin were beautiful because they were associated with Western civilisation: the catch-22 was that these features also 'proved' that white Western women were more beautiful than everybody else. Yet again, Western Europe became the normal standard by which everything was judged.

This was not just about aesthetic ideals. Beauty was also important to Victorians because personality was thought to be visible on the face. According to the science of physiognomy, introduced by the Swiss writer, philosopher and

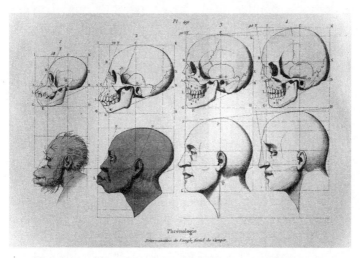

Petrus Camper's facial angle of 'beauty' depicted as a racist hierarchy of evolution, from Guerin's *Dictionnaire pittoresque d'histoire naturelle et des phénomènes de la nature, c.*1830.

theologian Johann Kaspar Lavater in 1775, the facial features indicated the character of the individual. By the later nineteenth century this was thought to reveal hereditary tendencies as well as individual inclinations. American physiognomist Samuel R. Wells, for example, offered up a number of unflattering portraits of women which reveal stark judgements about race and class.

In Wells's books, the popular icon of female beauty, Princess Alexandra of Denmark – who married Queen Victoria's eldest son in 1863 – was contrasted with the face of 'Sally Muggins', who, as her name suggests, was a generic simpleton of Celtic ancestry. Florence Nightingale – also an ideal of Western femininity – was contrasted with an Irish stereotype, with the similarly unflattering fictitious name of 'Bridget McBruiser'. Nightingale, drawn with wider eyes, rounder cheeks, and a straighter nose than her photographs attest to, is the ideal female face in contrast to McBruiser's flat nose, squinting eyes and sunken cheeks. Unlike Nightingale, McBruiser 'lives in the basement mentally as well as bodily', with every visible and invisible quality opposed to beauty: 'rude, rough, unpolished, ignorant, and brutish'.[17]

Wells was not alone in his derogatory attitude to Irish people. English writer and social reformer Charles Kingsley wrote of a visit to Ireland in July 1860 that he was 'haunted by the human chimpanzees I saw along that hundred miles of horrible country'. Despite their appearance, Kingsley claimed, Irish people were 'happier, better, more comfortably fed and lodged' under English rule.[18] Yet again we have supposed physical inferiority linked to justification for the 'benevolent' rule of wealthy colonisers (which conveniently

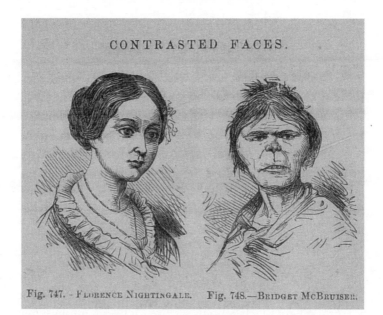

Caricature of 'Bridget McBruiser' as an unflattering comparison to Florence Nightingale in Samuel Wells's *New Physiognomy* (1867).

ignores the English failures and neglect during the recent Great Famine, which had flung so many people in Ireland into poverty and starvation). If the 'chimpanzees' had been Black, Kingsley went on in forthrightly racist tones, 'one would not feel it so much'.

Our idea of what is beautiful and what is normal appearance – and the link between the two – has certainly altered since the late Victorian era. Most of us don't feel we have been bred like racehorses or look for the ideal facial angle, and probably think it quite uncontroversial to sit upstairs on the omnibus or cut our hair short, as the Victorian 'New Woman' scandalously did. Cultural ideas of beauty have also shifted. In 1999, India became the beauty superpower of the world. Five Indian women won the pageants 'Miss Universe' and 'Miss World' between 1994 and 2000, and a new beauty industry emerged in South Asia.[19]

Yet today's standards of beauty continue to glorify a white body size and shape. Indian models have become thinner in search of the 'skinny white norm'.[20] In South Korea – the cosmetic surgery capital of the world – skin-lightening creams and surgery have become big business, as young women bleach their faces to an 'ideal' whiteness. And, across the Western world, women continue to alter their bodies at a higher rate than men through make-up, cosmetic surgery or dieting. Indeed, studies have shown that this increase has been especially marked for women of colour, who are more concerned about their body shape and size than their mothers and grandmothers were.[21] When Black schoolgirls are still sent home from schools for wearing natural hair – not straightened into the white ideal – it is a stark reminder of the colonial legacy that continues to infiltrate Western ideals of appearance.[22] Two centuries of scientific racism set white women up as the standard of beauty, a cultural practice that continues, often unconsciously, today.

FAT AND FIT

Some years ago, I worked on a project with a mental health arts group, reinterpreting objects in the Science Museum galleries through public tours. The personal stories stayed with me. I remember one gentleman, Peter, speaking in a gallery that dealt with nutrition and health. Peter described how he used to be a marathon runner. Since taking anti-depressants he had gained a lot of weight. Now, people in the street made judgements about him based on his appearance. 'Do you *really* need to eat that?' a complete stranger rudely demanded when Peter opened a chocolate bar while waiting for his train home one day. 'Try going on a diet!' someone else remarked when he arrived on the platform out of breath.

Peter's words struck me because I too had noticed the effect of antidepressants on my size. Looking back, I can probably name the medication I was taking at any given point based on my appearance in photographs. Sudden weight gain and puffy face? That'll be mirtazapine. Equally rapid weight loss and blotchy skin? Reboxetine, thank you very much. When my GP first prescribed mirtazapine to help with insomnia, he spoke rather dismissively of the weight gain that was a common side effect: 'If you exercise and eat healthily, you'll be fine.' I continued to religiously do the exact same exercise video I've followed since I was nine-teen years old (I am a creature of habit) and eat the same vaguely balanced diet of the twenty-something Londoner. I put on two stone. Anti-psychotic drugs have even more of an effect on weight than antidepressants. Oddly, despite this knowledge, the idea that weight might be related to factors beyond individual willpower had not really crossed my mind until I listened to Peter's talk. I grew up absorbing the fat stigma that pervades Western society without even really noticing it.

What has fat got to do with being normal, you might ask? Well, everything and nothing. The attitude towards larger people in Western society has shifted markedly over the last two centuries. In the eighteenth century, to be fat was unusual but desirable (a marker of wealth). Today, it is usual but undesirable (a sign of ill health). In both cases 'fatness' can be considered *either* normal or abnormal, depending on how you define the term. Attitudes to thinness have also changed. For Victorian women, a tiny waist was desirable – and achievable with tightly laced corsets – but a gaunt face suggested disease or poverty. Today, the thin, toned body is considered a symbol of success, the unachievable myth of the efficient businesswoman who exists on her drive alone – no sustenance needed!

When we talk about 'normal weight' today, we tend to think of an ideal, rather than what is usual. But how do we decide what is, in fact, optimal? The statistical study of weight goes all the way back to Adolphe Quetelet. Extraordinarily, the body mass index (BMI), widely used today to identify the healthy weight for a given height, relies on an equation devised by Quetelet in 1832. For many decades it was known as the Quetelet index. Quetelet divided weight in kilograms by height in metres squared to make the relationship between height and weight comparable across populations. He was not interested in obesity, but in human development. His archive includes an entire folder of the annual height and weight of his grandchildren Cécile, Marie and Juliette (his daughter Marie's children). What, he asked, was the expected height and weight at a given age?

Quetelet assumed that it was natural for weight to increase with age until a certain point in adult life when the wastage of old age set in. Even so, there was a huge variation in the figures the statistician used to obtain his averages. 'The extreme limits of the weight of well-formed individuals' ranged from 49.1 to 98.5 kg (7 st 10 lb to 15 st 7 lb) for men and 39.8 to 93.8 kg (6 st 4 lb to 14 st 11 lb) for women.[23] While the upper and lower measures were certainly a long way from the average, these men and women were still described as 'well-formed' and thus, presumably, normal. Not all Quetelet's subjects would be considered healthy according to today's use of his index. Even if we assume the tallest woman weighed the most – not necessarily the case – at 5 foot 8 she would have a BMI of 31.3, officially obese. But if Quetelet didn't draw such conclusions, where did this link between his formula and a healthy weight come from?

It was not until 1972 – well over a century later – that a group of researchers popularised the Quetelet index, renaming it the body mass index in the process.[24] This new name also changed the purpose of the formula. Quetelet's equation was only supposed to make it possible to compare large sets of data, not to judge individual people. By using the term 'body mass', Ancel Keys and his colleagues made the equation instead descriptive of individual bodies. Since then, this measure has remained the most popular way of determining physical health, although the boundaries of what is healthy have continued to shift, largely in favour of lower weights. When first introduced, a healthy BMI was regarded as $20–30 \text{ kg/m}^2$. Today, it is $18.5–25 \text{ kg/m}^2$, a considerable reduction.

We have something of a leap here. The body mass index moved from a descriptive measure of populations in 1832 to an index of healthy weight in 1972. How did this happen? Who decided what was a normal weight and how it related to health? Changing cultural expectations played a considerable role. As Amy Erdman Farrell's cultural history of fat shame shows, negative tropes about fat people long predated any link between excess weight and health. In fact, it was quite the reverse. As being overweight came to be seen as unhealthy towards the end of the Victorian period, pre-existing stereotypes about the lazy, greedy, primitive fat person were incorporated into a new medical model of physical health.[25]

Today, fat is often associated with a poor diet resulting from poverty. While this seems to acknowledge that healthier food is often more expensive, the unpleasant stereotype of the lazy couch potato is also widespread – think Harry Enfield's Wayne and Waynetta Slob, the 1990s comedy couple who spent their days slumped on the sofa in dirty, food-stained clothing. In the late nineteenth century, negative stereotypes linked to abnormal size were more often visited on the newly well-off middle classes. Unable to manage their newfound prosperity, the waists of the nouveau riche gradually expanded; or so thought the supposedly svelte upper classes.[26] Doctors, in contrast, continued to define weight gain as natural throughout a person's lifespan. Wasting diseases, like tuberculosis, were common, so putting on weight was often read as a sign of health. The American physician Silas Weir Mitchell's infamous rest cure for nervous diseases, first published in 1877, had the arresting title *Fat and Blood and How to Make Them*. Mitchell claimed that 'to gain in fat is nearly always to gain in blood' – i.e. healthy – and his regime of enforced bed rest and endless glasses of milk was designed to cure nervous symptoms by increasing both.[27]

As negative attitudes to weight grew, middle-class people became increasingly worried about their size. Diet guru William Banting tapped into popular concern about corpulence to publicise his own diet plan in 1880. 'When a corpulent man eats, drinks and sleeps well, has no pain to complain of and no particular organic disease, the judgement of able men seems paralyzed,' Banting complained.[28] While doctors thought an absence of pathological symptoms indicated a state of health, Banting disagreed. 'Banting' (the diet) became all the rage in late Victorian Britain. A bit like a Victorian version of the Atkins diet – which appeared a century or more later – it consisted largely of meat, though perhaps with a little more claret than its later equivalent.

The new diet industry at the turn of the twentieth century capitalised on the growing obsession with normal appearance. Diet pills and remedies proliferated from the late nineteenth century, becoming especially popular in the 1920s when a thin, flat-chested female body became the new normal. Adverts for these products highlighted the need for consumers to fit in. 'Obesity is an abnormal condition,' warned an 1878 advert for Allan's Anti-fat, an American vegetable remedy which claimed to prevent the body converting food into fat.[29] The 'Magic Figure Mold Garment', meanwhile, promised in 1914 to 'reduce abnormalities': 'If you are fat or ... if your figure is in any way abnormal, you need the Magic Figure Mold Garment.'[30] By the interwar period, the medical profession were starting to agree. 'To be built on the lines of a watermelon is no part of nature's plan for her highest creation,' admonished William Howard Hay, MD, in 1936.

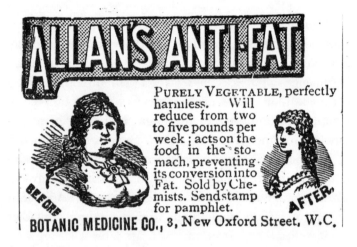

Late nineteenth-century advert for Allan's Anti-Fat, with 'before' and 'after' illustrations implying an increase in propriety alongside a decrease in weight from the buxom, matronly figure on the left to the girlish portrait on the right.

'Obesity is so unnecessary that the victim is to be regarded as one who is far from the normal.'[31] Fatness, and not the presence of disease, was a new way of defining the unhealthy abnormal body.

This hatred of fat was fixated on race as well as class. 'Are our women scrawny?' asked US fashion magazine *Harper's Bazaar* in 1896, concluding that no, white American slenderness was a positive trait since 'stoutness, corpulence, surplusage of flesh' was desirable only 'among African savages'.[32] As sociologist Sabrina Strings argues in *Fearing the Black Body*, in the eighteenth and early nineteenth centuries, the classification systems of 'race science' newly described European and African bodies in terms of physical difference, often focusing on size. These claims about size and weight were used to support the enslavement of African peoples by casting so-called gluttony as the opposite of reason.

Black people, the French naturalist Julien-Joseph Virey claimed in 1837, 'have a stupid look; they know of nothing but good eating; always digesting, they become incapable of thinking'.[33] Virey subscribed to the anthropological theory of 'polygenism', a widespread belief in early nineteenth-century science that human races descended from different origins. Yet even as 'monogenism' (the origin of the human species in one common ancestor) became dominant in evolutionary science, the distinctions between contemporary races made by polygenists like Virey continued to prove popular. Thus where certain groups, like the so-called 'Hottentots' of South Africa (a name given by Dutch colonists to the Khoikhoi people), were described as slender by eighteenth-century travellers, in the early nineteenth century, as 'fatness' became emphasised as a 'primitive' trait, the same people were recharacterised as fat.[34] Fatness, then, could be judged not by one's actual physical size and shape but by whether or not you belonged to a certain group, and was as much about race, class, power and control as the actual numbers on the scales.

But how were doctors to judge the boundaries of obesity? From the start, this decision was based entirely on comparison to others. Normal size, when it first emerged, was calculated from the average weight of one's fellow citizens, through the charts of the burgeoning insurance industry. Insurance companies, of course, were concerned with financial outcomes, not the health of an individual. Their weight, height and blood pressure tables aimed to exclude those with a potentially greater risk of dying from obtaining life insurance and ensure that lower premiums were given to people less likely to claim on their insurance.

It didn't matter that plenty of high-risk individuals did *not* die sooner than those considered lower risk, so long as the company made a profit. Since these companies helpfully collected large amounts of data, their figures became the statistics on which medical guides were based. Early tables for normal weight, then, simply used the average of the population at each height as a guide – or rather, the average of those who bought life insurance, who tended to be overwhelmingly white.

The first tables produced in the US by the Metropolitan Life Insurance Company (MLIC) in 1912 were used by doctors, nurses and nutritionists for decades. Around the same time as the tables were published, weighing scales began to appear in private homes, following their availability in shops in 1891.[35] When the MLIC published new data in 1942–3, they had transformed the average into an 'ideal' weight, as they now called it, based on the longevity of some 4 million policy holders. Yet MLIC's researchers encountered a problem. They couldn't fit their data into a normal distribution.[36] Well, not until they divided it not only by gender, age and height, but also into three different body frame sizes. This indicates how powerful the idea of the normal distribution was – the data was only persuasive when it fitted this model, even if that meant tinkering with the categories! It was never made clear how an ordinary person – or their doctor – was supposed to determine frame size. People had to fit the categories created by the data, and not the other way around. And this was the case whether they had been included in the calculations or not – essentially meaning that Black and Hispanic Americans had to conform to averages created from white bodies.

Medical concern about weight and health increased considerably from the 1950s, largely due to the connection between normal weight and normal blood pressure. This was highlighted by the 1959 Build and Blood Pressure Study, carried out in the US by the Society of Actuaries, and influential across the Western world. The study claimed to link obesity, high blood pressure and high mortality, based on a huge survey of 4.9 million insurance policies. It wasn't the first time these things had been connected: indeed, the introduction to the study notes that it was undertaken in the belief that the traits were linked, and that deaths from obesity and high blood pressure had risen in recent years.[37] The study generated data that shaped ideas of healthy sizes for decades afterwards. Despite this, the definition of overweight was, once again, calculated on the average. An overweight person was someone who weighed 10 per cent more than the average person, and a very overweight person weighed 20 per cent more.

The body mass index was supposed to do away with averages, by applying a simple, objective calculation to all. This, Keys assumed, would help to get rid of 'disgusting' and 'repugnant' obesity, emphasising the ongoing negativity associated with fatness.[38] Yet it is well known that BMI cannot deal with the bodies of certain athletes – rugby players, for example – since a simple calculation cannot differentiate between fat and muscle. It also cannot take into account that Black people tend to have a higher muscle mass and bone density than white people.[39] Just like its predecessor, BMI is not a definitive measure of health: it doesn't measure our fitness levels or circumstances. Some overweight people in the MLIC tables did not have a greater mortality risk than thinner people, even if some of them did. Similarly, not everyone with a BMI in the obese range will be unhealthy, even if some are. One 2003 study indicated that Black women aren't at significant risk of reduced life expectancy until they reach a BMI of 37.[40] Yet the history of this particular normal standard – the skinny white ideal – reveals how generations of people have been stigmatised because their body shape did not meet certain culturally determined criteria.

LESS THAN ZERO

All my life, I've heard friends bemoan the challenges of clothes shopping. One can't buy knee-high boots, because her calves are larger than the average. Another used to buy trousers two waist sizes too big for her, because otherwise they never reached her ankles. Others complain about the width of sleeves or tiny bust sizes in high-street shops – 'they're made for flat-chested teenagers!' When a multitude of measurements make up any one item of clothing, it's a wonder we ever find anything to fit us at all.

The rise of a consumer society has exacerbated the challenges of being a 'normal' size. Before the late nineteenth century, most people made their own clothes, or had them tailored to fit. In 1880s London, anatomist's daughter Jeanette Marshall spent much of her time sewing: making, altering and embellishing gowns for dances and events.[41] Even in 1918, Virginia Woolf complained that her sister Vanessa ignored a performance Virginia and Roger Fry put on at Charleston, because she was 'sitting almost silent, stitching a dress by lamplight'.[42]

Mass markets gave us the simplicity of off-the-peg outfits, which required the individual to fit the cloth-ing rather than the other way around. This began with uniforms, first in the army where large quantities were needed. Officers found themselves frustrated with the stan-dard sizes provided. 'I would here again state (as I have often before in previous reports)', complained US Colonel George Croghan in his report of August 1831, 'that very many of the pantaloons issued to the soldiers are too small and short.'[43] Nonetheless, ready-to-wear clothing was con-venient, and men's coats and suits became more widely available, with sizes often determined using statistics from the very same military. By 1847, ready-to-wear clothing was made by 233 different manufacturers in Paris. In New York, Brooks Brothers, founded by Henry Brooks in 1818, intro-duced ready-to-wear suits in 1849.

According to historian Robert Ross, the popularity of these items was largely down to marketing.[44] In an 1860 promotional brochure, London firm E. Moses and Son was one of many to lay claim to being 'the first House in London or, we may say, in the World, that established the system of NEW CLOTHING READY-MADE'. This advertising was designed to appeal to the fast pace of modern life, linking off-the-peg suits with technologi-cal progress: 'Tailoring is as rapid in these days as railway travelling.' Eighty per cent of British men were now buying ready-made clothing, E. Moses claimed, probably exagger-atedly (they actually said 'of the population', but men were after all the norm).[45]

Western-style clothing quickly spread around the world. Between 1880 and 1950, Ross claims, Africa saw a 'virtually complete reclothing of half a continent'.[46] While some city dwellers in Sierra Leone, Ghana and Nigeria had been buying suits and frock coats from London tailors since the 1860s, ready-to-wear clothing met increased demand in these countries. Elsewhere, too, suits replaced traditional clothing. In 1872, the Japanese government declared that Western clothing was compulsory for male government officials (which soon after spread to businesses and schools), while the founder of the new Turkey, Kemal Atatürk, proclaimed in 1925 that 'a civilized, international dress is worthy and appropriate for our nation, and we will wear it'.[47] Not only was the suit now produced in a set range of sizes, but it had become the global norm.

Interestingly, women's clothing continued to vary by country. Even as increasing numbers of men dressed in identical three-piece suits, Japanese women still wore kimonos, and the sari remained popular across India. And in Europe many women wore home-made or tailored clothing until the middle of the twentieth century. In Chester in 1944, a survey showed that many women were still making their own dresses and knitwear, or paying a dressmaker to do so.[48]

Norma re-enters the story here: the average American statue of 1945 was created from the measurements of 14,698 white US citizens gathered by the Bureau of Home Economics in 1940 to try to create the first standardised system of sizing for women's ready-made clothing.[49] The final report struggled to decide exactly which out of the fifty-eight body measurements taken could be used to create set sizes, but focused on 'weight, stature, bust girth, waist girth and hip girth'. This is not to say that other measurements did not vary but, after all, 'maximum thigh girth would be inconvenient to take on a full-clothed woman'.[50] Bust, waist and hips became the key measurements for women's clothing and remain so to this day. If, like me, you've ever had to buy trousers that are loose around the waist in order to squeeze them over your thighs, you might find yourself frustrated by this decision.

From the 1950s, mass-produced clothing became the norm, with Norma's measurements replaced by a wider study of American women which created a sizing system ranging from 8 to 38 with variations for different body types (as with the Build and Blood Pressure studies, this notion of diverse body types is something we have mysteriously lost over the years). This meant that not only did women's bodies have to fit into a specific set of averages at every stage, but a maximum limit on the size of normal bodies was set: the largest commercially available size. And while the assigned size numbers were rather arbitrary, as women became used to interpreting these figures dress manufacturers realised that their clothing would be more popular if people were able to buy smaller sizes. Accordingly, the measurements associated with each size grew – and began to vary considerably between suppliers, making truly standard sizing a thing of the past.

Clothing sizes also vary by country, of course. I remember being immensely confused when the size zero furore hit the press in the early 2000s. Size zero was blamed for a decline in female body image and a rise in eating disorders, especially after the death of Uruguayan model

Luisel Ramos in 2006. Since the smallest clothes in UK high-street shops were a size 8 (with the very occasional 6), I couldn't work out where this 0 came from or how it was physically possible for anyone to be that small. It turned out a 0 actually was that occasional 6. A UK women's size 14 is often a 10 in the US, a 40 in Germany, a 46 in Italy and a 66 in Korea. And when it comes to small, medium and large, in this age of globally available clothing, no one knows what to buy!

Finally, remember the lesson of Norma. While her statistics may have come from averages generated for the first standardised clothing sizes, in the end not one single woman measured up to the statue. A size 14 blouse is tailored to everyone and no one at the same time. So what are the chances you'd actually fit into it anyway?

ADDITIONAL CHARMS OF PERSON

On 6 January 1899, London's Olympia hosted an 'indignation meeting'. It was called by Annie Jones, the daughter of one of the First Families of Virginia and a performer in Barnum and Bailey's 'Greatest Show on Earth'. The show was in London for the second time in a Europe-wide tour, which had begun in 1897. It boasted performing animals, acrobats, aerial and horseback displays and what was then popularly known as a freakshow. Annie Jones had prepared a series of resolutions against this description of the 'human abnormalities and specialty artists' within the show. 'Freak', Miss Jones complained, meant something like 'fright'. This made no sense when applied to people. If a beard such as hers made a lady a fright, Jones concluded, then the same must apply to a man – and no man possessing as fine a beard as she did would ever consider himself a fright! Newspapers reported that every member of the assembly supported the motion.

The performers concluded that the word freak was an indignity, unjustly conferred because, 'fortunately or otherwise, we are possessed with more or less limbs, more or less hair, more or less bodies, more or less physical or mental attributes than other people'. These attributes, Annie Jones held, were not frightful or abnormal but 'additional charms of person or aids to movement'. Further, 'in the opinion of many, some of us are really the development of a higher type, and are superior persons, inasmuch as some of us are gifted with extraordinary attributes not apparent in ordinary beings'.[51] Freakishness is all a matter of perspective.

The week after the 'revolt of the freaks' – as newspapers termed the meeting – the group met again to vote on an alternative name. Nearly a dozen were suggested, although most, like 'paradox' and 'curio', received just one vote apiece. 'Human marvel' was popular, but 'prodigy' stormed into the lead with twenty-one votes.[52] Both terms reflected the extraordinary attributes claimed by the performers. Yet both were also, perhaps, slightly closer to the word 'freak' than we might today imagine. Adverts for the Greatest Show on Earth referred to the team as 'the famous collection of wonderful freaks'. Like the performing elephants in this travelling circus, 'freaks' were exhibited as wonders of nature.

The heyday of the freakshow ran from the 1840s well

into the twentieth century. As disability historian Rose-marie Garland-Thomson explains, someone was not born a freak. The freak was created from the 'ordinary other' through staging, costume, the spiel of the pitchman, care-fully crafted background narratives and expert testimony.[53] The abnormal body was just as much a product of context and attitudes as the normal. No distinction was made between congenital difference and self-embellishment: the 'armless wonder' and the 'tattooed lady' were equally freakish. Colonialism and the increasing popularity of evo-lutionary theory made ethnicity a key boundary played on by freakshows in the later nineteenth century:[54] from the 'Egyptian juggler', 'whirling dervishes' and 'head-swinging Soudanese' to Jo-Jo the Dog-Faced Boy (Fedor Adri-anovich Jeftichew), who liked to read 'tales of adventure in Russian'.[55] The back story was nearly as important as appearance, even when it was entirely invented. Pip and Flip, the 'twins from Yucatan' in the World Circus Side Show, were actually born Jenny and Elvira Snow in the state of Georgia.[56]

As evolutionary theory took hold, show bills began to present some prodigies as the 'missing link' between human and ape, a popular illustration of Darwinism. A sideshow act presented by showman P. T. Barnum, co-founder of the 'Greatest Show on Earth', called 'What Is It?' was supposed to be man's evolutionary ancestor, found by Bar-num's representatives in some unspecified place in Africa. From at least 1877, however, the role was played by a Black American man with learning disabilities.[57] Showpieces like this played on scientific racism that claimed that people of colour were less evolved than white people. Shows increasingly exhibited – and exploited – non-Western people transported to America and Europe by explorers, missionaries and scientists, while some prodigies were also enslaved African Americans.* After appearing at the 1904 Saint Louis World's Fair, a Congolese Mbuti man named Ota Benga was even displayed in the monkey house at the Bronx Zoo, sharing a space with a trained orangutan named Dohong. African American community leaders protested Ota Benga's exhibition as racist. Most, however, also took care to set themselves apart from a man they described as an uncivilised African 'boy', very different from the educated Black American.[58]

The Olympia indignation meeting shows that some performers were starting to reclaim their difference. By the turn of the twentieth century, however, the scientific view prevailed – and the sometimes celebrated, sometimes exploited differences of prodigies and performers became simply medical aberrations to be addressed. Normal standards grew increasingly narrow and prescriptive, as the chilling epigraph added by the distributor to Tod Browning's 1932 film *Freaks* put it: 'Never again will such a story be filmed ... as modern science and teratology is rapidly eliminating such blunders of nature from the world.'[59]

Bodily difference was becoming something to be either 'fixed' or hidden away. At the same time as 'freaks' were marvelled at on stage, disabled bodies were disappearing from the streets of America, forced behind closed doors, or into ungainly – but visually acceptable – prosthetics by

* P. T. Barnum's first performer was Joice Heth, purchased by the entertainer in 1835 as (supposedly) George Washington's former nursemaid, now aged 161.

so-called 'ugly laws' that targeted those who were physically different.

Historian Susan Schweik has charted the history of these laws – sometimes thought to be an urban myth – across a variety of US states and cities from 1867 until the last documented arrest in Omaha, Nebraska, in 1974.[60] In this final, unexpectedly late example, a police officer arrested a homeless man because he had 'marks and scars' on his body, but the city prosecutors questioned the definition of ugliness and the case was dropped.[61] While 'ugly laws' framed disabled bodies as both abnormal and unpleasant, they focused mainly on begging. Disabled beggars, street musicians and salespeople were thought to be a public nuisance because of their unusual bodies *and* their working practices. 'Unsightly beggar ordinances' found their way into English and German newspapers too, if not necessarily the law.[62]

Yet, paradoxically, increasing numbers of people *were* physically different from others, thanks to the twin hazards of industrialisation and war. 'It is not two years since the sight of a person who had lost one of his lower limbs was an infrequent occurrence,' American physician and poet Oliver Wendell Holmes noted in 1863. 'Now, alas! there are few of us who have not a cripple among our friends, if not in our own families.'[63] As physical difference became more usual, however, it became more stigmatised. The disabled beggar was 'an unsightly or disgusting object', Chicago laws of 1881 announced, determining to rid the streets of these supposedly corrupting influences.[64] From 1867, when the earliest statute was passed in San Francisco, to 1905 when Reno, Nevada, joined the ranks, 'ugly laws' were passed in a range of US cities, and even across the entire

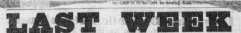
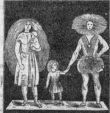
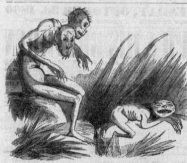

Flyer for a P. T. Barnum show, emphasising the way 'freakshows' built on racist interpretations of evolutionary science, 1860.

state of Pennsylvania in 1891.[65]

Although police often ignored the statutes, some disabled people lost their livelihoods as a result. One young man born with clubbed hands and feet, the son of poor Polish immigrants, grew up dependent on his siblings to carry him around. At sixteen he began 'the only kind of work that seemed possible' – selling newspapers on street corners. His life was straightforward until his job was abolished by 'the enforcement of a statute that prevented cripples from exposing their deformity by selling on street corners'.* Luckily, a friendly druggist allowed the young man to use his doorway and, when interviewed by an investigator from the Welfare Federation of Cleveland in 1916, the 'fine-looking' thirty-five-year-old was still selling papers, happy with his work, and had no interest in medical intervention. 'My life,' he told the investigator, 'is satisfactory to me as it is.'[66]

This young man's attitude would not have been acceptable in 'polite society', where it was expected that disability would be covered up. 'Misfortunes of a certain obtrusiveness may be pitied,' Oliver Wendell Holmes reflected, 'but are never tolerated under the chandeliers.'[67] This wasn't just in the US. Across the Western world, from the UK to Western Russia, prosthetics were designed for appearance as much as function during the nineteenth and twentieth centuries.[68] To be disabled was only acceptable if it was hidden. The Welfare Federation of Cleveland claimed proudly that the 'capacity, occupations, and earnings [of disabled people] point on the whole to varied and normal tendencies of

* It is unclear exactly when this statute was passed in Cleveland: it is not specified in the source, nor did Schweik find a date in her research.

life'.[69] Rather than society adapting to the needs of the individual, it was considered the disabled person's responsibility to conceal or overcome their 'abnormality'.

Yet most did not find life as easy or straightforward as the Cleveland survey concluded. In Birmingham, England, in 1911, only 20 per cent of physically disabled men were in work, and their wages were low.[70] The increasing possibility of medical intervention did not, then, make disabled bodies any more accepted in the workforce. In North America in particular, the assumption that a combination of medicine and hard work could allow anyone to transcend disability actually increased negative attitudes towards many disabled people. Punitive attempts to 'normalise' those who were different occurred in other countries too. In Britain, Deaf children were discouraged from using British Sign Language – and even punished for doing so – until the 1970s. Only in 2003 did BSL become classed as a minority language. And we are living with the hangover of these attitudes and acts of exclusion today: almost 43 per cent of disabled people in the UK are economically inactive, compared to only about 15 per cent of non-disabled, while austerity and welfare cuts have hit disabled people particularly hard.* This hostility was epitomised in the attitude of the government to the 'vulnerable' during the first waves of Covid-19, which led to disproportionate deaths among the disabled community (six out of ten people who died from Covid-19 in the UK in 2020 were disabled).[71]

The demand to fit in can also be a heavy burden. Perhaps the most famous example of someone who

* In 2017 a UN Committee expressed grave concerns about the UK government's failure to uphold the rights of disabled people during a period of austerity.

supposedly 'transcended' their disability is US president Franklin D. Roosevelt (1882–1945). Roosevelt, like so many others around the world, was severely disabled by polio. Although famous as a polio survivor in his lifetime, Roosevelt carefully hid the extent of his disability. The politician was never pictured in a wheelchair (despite using one) and would be secretly carried into inaccessible venues up back stairs or enter supported by bodyguards to make it appear that he was walking. Roosevelt himself regarded disability as a sign of weakness, in a political leader at least. Crutches, he thought, inspired 'fear, revulsion and pity', and he determined to 'stand easily enough in front of people so that they'll forget I'm a cripple'.[72] It was not until 1994, fifty years after his death, that the extent of Roosevelt's disability became publicly known.[73]

The myth that Roosevelt created, exacerbated by the American ideals of self-sufficiency and individual achievement, left many other polio survivors in the US with an impossible act to follow. Doctors, families and therapists urged other patients to follow Roosevelt's example. Polio survivors 'passing in the shadow of FDR' adopted a range of strategies to hide the visible effects of polio and 'pass as normal'.[74] This could have serious consequences, from the physical damage caused by walking instead of using a wheelchair to the emotional strain of emulating others. American high-school student and polio survivor Stanley Lipshultz 'pretended to be normal and kept up with the best of them'. It was only later in life that Lipshultz reflected that 'passing, unfortunately, came with a price'. 'Who knew?' Lipshultz wondered. 'Being "normal" took an enormous amount of energy, both physical and emotional.'[75]

WHAT IS A NORMAL BODY?

When I was in my late twenties, I worked for a short time in a university public engagement team. We ran events and training to help academics talk to other people about their research – not always an easy task. Until then, I'd never really considered how inaccessible many public and educational institutions were. After all, I'd never had to. One of my colleagues used a wheelchair, and I accompanied her on a trip around campus, inspecting potential rooms for our events. All the places we visited were listed as wheelchair accessible. But, as I quickly found out, this did not mean it was true. We took back-lifts and meandered down corridors I'd never seen before, encountering obstacles with no seeming purpose other than to frustrate us in our journey. I marvelled at the amount of time my colleague had to waste checking something the institution ought simply to provide. She shrugged, surprisingly tolerantly; she was used to it. For her it was a daily necessity.

The experience stuck with me as I pushed my way through furious hordes of racing commuters on the Tube journey home. I wondered how the people tutting at the two-minute delay to their train would cope with the time added to their journey if they needed to traipse down an extra corridor to reach the lift. Stepping off a pavement outside, I didn't even look for the nearest dropped kerb. But the London Borough of Westminster, a friend tells me, is a nightmare for wheelchair users because of a serious lack of them. Your journey from one place to another might double – triple even – from all the back and forth needed just to cross a road. And this is decades after the first Disability Discrimination Act in the UK (1995) and nearly fifty years after the social model of disability was first outlined.

The history of the 'normal' body as seen through the treatment and understanding of disability is often controversial, and usually disturbing. In the nineteenth and early twentieth centuries narratives of disability veered between the 'marvels' of freakshow displays and inspirational stories of overcoming adversity. In this era the 'ugly laws' merged almost seamlessly into a narrative of medical improvement. There was no question of society accommodating difference: the individual was expected to overcome or at the very least conceal any unusual physical traits.

While some prodigies – like those who held their indignation meeting in 1899 – had long been questioning the way they were viewed, it was not until much later that such exclusion began to be questioned on a wider level. The social model of disability was nicely summed up for me in a conversation I had a few years ago with artist and activist Penny Pepper. 'Some say "people with disabilities",' she told me; 'I prefer "disabled people" because it gets across the message that disabilities are not something we have. We are disabled *by* society.' When disabled activists developed the idea in the late 1970s, the social model of disability turned the individualised medical model of normality on its head, insisting that society, not disabled people, was required to change.

Indeed, while normal has often been assumed to be an ability to look and function like everyone else, to fit in is not necessarily optimal. In 1906, George Bernard Shaw had his eyes tested by a physician friend, who described the playwright's sight as 'normal'. When Shaw 'naturally took this to mean it was like everybody else's' his friend 'hastened to explain to me that I was an exceptional and highly fortunate person optically'. Only 10 per cent of the population, Shaw's friend explained, had perfect vision; fully 90 per cent were abnormal.[76] Shaw was gifted with an ability not present in ordinary individuals. Yet would any of us class someone who doesn't wear glasses as abnormal?[77] If not, why not?

Perfect eyesight, like a perfect body, is an ideal almost everyone fails to live up to. None of us, after all, are Norma or Normman, average man or woman. Yet the individual model that has prevailed for much of the twentieth century makes us view our differences from the average as a personal failing. We lament our inability to squeeze into a pair of trousers with a 32-inch waist, while never considering the multitude of hidden measurements that go into a single piece of clothing. Maybe we *are* a 32-inch waist after all, we just don't have the average thigh or calf or leg length that corresponds to it. When military engineers measured pilots against the average sizes used in cockpits in the 1940s, they found that not a single pilot out of 4,063 fell in the average range in all ten dimensions used.[78]

So it's not only clothes that are the issue. My brother-in-law – considerably taller than average – struggles to find a bed long enough to suit him if he travels from home. When I helped to set up a work event about how to cut your own hair in lockdown, one colleague had a lot of experience to draw on because for years she had been unable to find a hairdresser who could cut and style afro-textured hair in her hometown in Wales. In a consumer society, everything is made to fit an average, from the normal height of a door handle and a light switch to the amount of salt in a ready meal. Not only are these averages unlikely to take into account the needs of those of us disabled by society, in actual fact they may be optimal for very few of us at all.

Throughout history, though, normal and abnormal bodies have always been about more than just the individual. Since the second half of the nineteenth century, the changing size, shape and appearance of bodies has been used to illustrate or justify wider fears. From degeneration to the 'obesity epidemic', average and exceptional bodies have been thought to signify national and social decline. The body has illustrated fears about industrial city life and moral decline, concern about failures in public health and excessive state involvement in society, the threat of the underclass, of feminism and racial mixing. Yet all these fears about difference relied on one underlying and often unacknowledged thing: the assumption about what was normal in the first place. This was the white, middle-class, usually male and never disabled body. This notion of an 'ideal' normalcy continues to underpin Western society to this day. Recognising its existence is the first step in taking it down.

3

DO I HAVE A
NORMAL MIND?

I stand in the empty hospital corridor for ten whole minutes, glancing from the rack of information leaflets to the
signs and posters. My eyes are repeatedly drawn back to the
visiting rules next to the locked, windowless door. Visiting
hours, I read, are 5–9 p.m. All visitors must leave the ward
by 9 p.m. It's now 6 p.m. It's fine.

Eventually I press the doorbell and a buzzer sounds,
the door unlocking to allow me into a small anteroom. A
woman is barely visible behind a glass screen; there is a
visitor book on a shelf in front of it. I tell her I'm here to
see my friend and she buzzes me through the second locked
door without a word. She doesn't ask me to sign in.

Inside, the corridor is wider but just as nondescript. I feel
confused and ever so slightly scared. I have no idea where
I'm supposed to go and there's no one to ask. Luckily, when
I turn to the right, I see my friend walking towards me. She
beams widely: she had no idea I was coming today, and it's
just chance that she was in the right place at the right time.
She is followed by a nurse, who glowers at me warily. My

friend hugs me and asks if there's somewhere we can talk. The nurse looks even more suspicious.

'Who is she?' she demands.

'Sarah is my friend!' my friend announces. Appeased by this explanation, the nurse lets us into a side room where we can sit and talk. I'm not sure who she thought I might be to greet me with such hostility.

The strangest part of visiting a friend in a locked psychiatric unit is the place itself. Compared to this, any eccentricities of the people inhabiting it pale into insignificance. After several visits, I concluded that the ward was designed to *drive* people mad. All information is placed only where it can't be accessed: the information leaflets outside the secure main doors, a poster explaining your right to see a mental health advocate in the locked staff toilet, which my friend persuades another uncertain staff member to let me use. Staff fail to answer the most basic of questions or push back on simple requests like a need to use the laundry room or charge a phone. Another patient points out the one-way window, which allows you to see into the admitting room from the corridor. 'I was in there all last night – you can't tell anyone's watching you from inside and no one tells you,' she says dismally. Residents slump vacantly on the sofa in front of the day room TV or smoke in the rooftop garden. No one bothers to enforce the No Smoking signs plastered everywhere.

As a lone visitor, I am gold dust. I am the one interesting thing to happen that evening, perhaps even that day or week. My friend and I sit in the weed-infested garden and person after person approaches to interrupt our conversation with elaborate tales of past lives, real and imagined.

As my first visit draws to a close, my friend and I go back to stand near the entrance. No one in the glassed-in office even looks our way. We ask another patient how to leave but she doesn't know. The minutes tick past. It's now half past nine, visiting hours are long over. I start to wonder: if I just stand here chatting, will I simply be absorbed into the mundane life of the ward? I never signed in, after all. Maybe I will never be allowed to leave.

Then a man appears at the window of the nurses' station, and my friend knocks on the glass.

'Can my friend leave?' she asks. The man looks at me for a long, appraising moment, and eventually he nods. We hug goodbye and she stands back so he will open the door.

My visit to a twenty-first-century psychiatric hospital reminded me of the famous 1970s psychology study 'On Being Sane in Insane Places'. 'If sanity and insanity exist, how shall we know them?' asked author David Rosenhan.[1] How indeed? The ward where I visited my friend, its rules and procedures, seemed frankly bizarre. And for centuries the 'madhouse' has also been an allegory for society, so much so that the name of the old Bethlem Royal Hospital – Bedlam – came to mean general chaos and unrest. The final scene in William Hogarth's morality tale *A Rake's Progress* shows Tom Rakewell confined in Bedlam, driven mad by his dissolute lifestyle. People often assume this is an exact depiction of the hospital in 1735. Yet the engraving can also be read, like most of Hogarth's works, as social commentary. One patient wears a crown and holds a sceptre, another worships a crucifix while two wealthy ladies come visiting. Religion, nationalism, politics

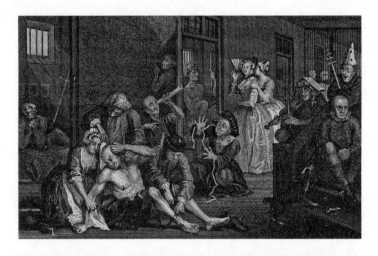

The final print (plate 8) in Hogarth's *A Rake's Progress*, showing Tom Rakewell (the 'rake' of the title) confined to Bedlam as a result of his drunken, dissolute lifestyle (1735–63).

and the class system may be just as crazy in the end as the madhouse itself.

Rosenhan's study has become one of the classics of psychology since it was first published in 1973. According to Rosenhan's report, eight 'pseudopatients' sought admission to a variety of psychiatric hospitals across five US states. All of them complained of hearing voices, often unclear, but repeating words like 'empty', 'hollow' and 'thud'. All eight were admitted to hospital, where most were diagnosed with schizophrenia and remained inpatients for between seven and fifty-two days. Although the participants, which included Rosenhan himself, were instructed to behave 'normally' after admission, none were detected as pseudopatients by staff – although their fellow inmates were often more suspicious. When discharged, most were not deemed cured but to have 'schizophrenia in remission'.

Many have questioned and disagreed with Rosenhan's study over the years – and even, more recently, wondered if he might have made most of his pseudopatients up.[2] Nonetheless, Rosenhan's conclusions inspired – and were inspired by – key figures in the anti-psychiatry movement of the 1960s and 1970s. People like R. D. Laing, David Cooper and Thomas Szasz – psychiatrists with very different backgrounds and beliefs – publicly questioned the institutions and practices of psychiatry. They also debated the idea of normalcy itself. 'Anxiety and depression exist. Psychological suffering exists,' Rosenhan clarified. 'But normality and abnormality, sanity and insanity, and the diagnoses that flow from them may be less substantive than many believe them to be.'[3]

Although the anti-psychiatry movement is often assumed to be the birth of uncertainty about the normal mind, David Rosenhan was hardly the first person in history who questioned the boundary between madness and sanity. The divide between the normal and abnormal mind – and if there is, in fact, any such thing – has been debated by psychiatrists, psychologists and, of course, their patients for at least the last 150 years. We may be even less certain about the normality of our minds than of our bodies, which at least give us tangible evidence of difference. After all, mental science has rarely – even in our era of neuroscience and brain scans – been able to provide biological or physiological evidence of the origins of any disorder, meaning that mental illness today – as it was in 1870 – is defined largely by unconventional behaviour and experiences. So, how do we decide what's normal and what isn't?

HEARING VOICES

Louis Box was plagued with doubts about the world around him. A young writer with a vivid imagination, Louis lived in a boarding house in Earl's Court. At least, he had thought it was a boarding house when he moved in. Now he was not so sure. It was December 1891. As Louis walked through the dark London streets, collar turned up against the bitter wind, detectives followed him. People sniffed as he passed by, and often Louis heard them make sarcastic remarks. 'He appears pretty happy this morning!' he heard someone sneer as he turned a corner one day. 'There he goes!' said another voice as Louis approached his home. He knew what these people meant. Everybody thought that Louis Box was Jack the Ripper, the murderer of East End women who had never been caught.

The boarding house, Louis realised, was in the pay of the police. Here, Louis was subjected to every kind of machination, with a view to making him confess to crimes he had not committed. The owner of the house was French, but Louis quickly realised that he was no ordinary Frenchman. This Earl's Court boarding house was run by none other than the famous neurologist Jean-Martin Charcot himself! Thinking Box was out of earshot one day, Charcot confessed to an accomplice that Louis had realised who he was, definite proof that the ageing neurologist had travelled to London to become a lodging-house landlord.

It was Charcot who set up the experiments designed to torture Louis Box into confessing. Box received shocks from wires in his bed. There were telephones in the room, and a false back to the cupboard. The writer heard Charcot discussing his earlier life with the police. Sometimes, the doctor would imitate the falling of drops of blood, watching Box intently to see what effect this had on him. At other times, the conspirators would flash lights before him and show Box indecent pictures. It was not improbable, Louis concluded, that Charcot had hypnotised him to see if he had homicidal tendencies.

Louis Box's tale sounds like the sort of ripping yarn one might find in a 1920s Boy's Own adventure annual. It was, however, the story of a young man admitted to Bethlem Royal Hospital in December 1891. The oldest psychiatric hospital in the country, Bethlem was founded in 1247. By Box's time, the charitable institution had moved twice from its original home in Bishopsgate, and now inhabited leafy grounds in Lambeth. Today, this building is London's Imperial War Museum (Bethlem moved again, for the final time, in 1930). It is a beautiful building with an ornate dome, where the hospital's wealthy governors claimed that the scandals that had once beset Bethlem were relics of a distant past. Public visiting, which aimed to encourage donations to the charitable institution, had been deemed inhumane and ended in 1770. In the early 1850s, metal and canvas restraints were removed from the wards. Nonetheless, the locked doors of the hospital remained an unwelcome confinement to many of its inhabitants. When one patient, known as Kentish Scribbler, sketched the hospital in the 1870s, she drew it as a birdcage; the doctor outside the cage held the only key.

Louis Box ended up in Bethlem when, frightened and depressed by the unrelenting persecution, he told his brother and several doctors that the only way out of his situation was suicide. Just because these people thought Louis was delusional did not make the experience any less distressing for Louis himself. Louis's story also weaves together many different elements of late Victorian psychology: the Whitechapel murders of 1888, experimental psychology, spiritualism and hypnosis, new technologies – electricity and the telephone – and even new understandings of the mind. Box eventually concluded that, although he had not consciously murdered anyone, he might have done so *un*consciously. As new psychological approaches to mind grew in importance, so too did the idea that not all actions were prompted by conscious thought: in the 1890s theories of the unconscious, subconscious and double consciousness were used to explain automatic behaviour or hidden memories.

It was supremely difficult for Louis Box to function 'normally' under such unpleasant circumstances. The world he was experiencing was not normal; indeed, his reactions to it might appear completely rational if we too believed he had been persecuted. This is something that former mental health nurse and novelist Nathan Filer points out to great effect in his 2019 non-fiction book on schizophrenia, *The Heartland*. Filer tells the stories of his interviewees exactly as they experienced them. 'It is the person,' Filer points out, that lies at the centre of psychiatry. 'It is their story.'[4] If you were sure that you were being experimented on by your landlord, I'm guessing that you too would be deeply distressed. Chances are this feeling would even survive an eventual realisation that the situation wasn't quite what you had thought it was.

This happened to me, fifteen years ago, during a stressful period at work. I sat in the library writing on my day off when I suddenly realised that two unknown women on the other side of the room were talking about me. I watched them carefully while pretending to work. I feigned indifference, getting up to search for a book on a slightly closer shelf. I could only catch one word in ten, but this didn't shake my conviction that they were spreading malicious rumours about me. Today, I'm pretty sure the work stress had made me paranoid. My memory of that moment, however, and the emotions accompanying it, is just as clear; I can even see the sidelong glances the women gave me, despite knowing they probably never happened.

The way we interpret and function in social situations is, to a large extent, a matter of perception. These perceptions themselves are shaped by biases and assumptions about what is normal, often based on class, race and gender. Yet 'abnormal behaviour' has often been the acid test for psychosis. 'Central to our concept of schizophrenia is the notion that the disorder interferes with normal social functioning,' the creators of the American psychiatric bible, the DSM-III, stated firmly in 1980,* rooting the diagnosis of serious mental illness in an inability to behave normally.[5] But how do we judge the extent of such interference? Or even what normal social functioning is in the first place? Both of these things tend to be based on our experiences of the world around us; these experiences will be different depending on the time or country in which we live, our

* DSM stands for 'Diagnostic and Statistical Manual of Mental Disorders', first published by the American Psychiatric Association (APA) in 1952. It is generally known by its initials and the edition (in Roman numerals for I–IV, switching to Arabic numerals for DSM-5). The current edition, DSM-5, was published in 2013.

age, gender, race and background. Normal functioning is not universal.

Perhaps Louis Box's fantastical life seems obviously abnormal to some readers, even if you can appreciate that it was entirely real to Louis himself. What, then, about the description of another, much more mundane, morning a few years earlier, in 1886? Mr Joseph Kirk of Ripon Villas, Plumstead, was halfway through dressing when he was startled by a loud bang. Kirk assumed the sound to be the latch-lock of the front basement door slamming closed and realised to his annoyance that the milkman must be late. This had been a frequent frustration recently, meaning Mary, the servant, had to go out and fetch milk before breakfast. Mr Kirk finished dressing and descended the stairs to the kitchen, passing Mary on the way. The girl was dressed in her outdoor clothes – a brown straw hat and black cloth jacket over her light print frock. As Kirk reached the kitchen door, Mary passed behind him towards the scullery. Still annoyed at the milkman, Mr Kirk voiced his frustration aloud to his wife: 'So Mary has had to go out for milk again.' Surprised, Kirk's wife shook her head. 'Mary has not been out this morning,' she told him firmly, 'and she is now in the breakfast-room at work.' Joseph Kirk realised that the Mary he had seen and heard must have been a 'very vivid and life-like hallucination'.[6]

Hallucinations – hearing or seeing things that others do not – are today widely viewed as serious symptoms of madness. Yet they are also a symptom of many other conditions: of fever, infection or drug-induced delirium. When my elderly mother-in-law began to see animals climbing up the walls and ethereal figures starting fires in her living room, my partner and I were at a loss, until antibiotics for a urinary infection resolved them entirely. Despite this, we had to repeatedly argue with GPs who refused to come out with a prescription when she next began hallucinating, alone and scared, miles away from where we live. 'There's nothing I can do,' said one doctor; 'it's dementia' – even though we knew it wasn't and told him so.

A sudden deterioration in eyesight can also cause hallucinations, known as Charles Bonnet Syndrome, as the brain tries to fill unexpected gaps in the information it receives from the optic nerve. And even what someone with twenty-twenty vision sees is not an objective picture of the world in front of them, but always filtered by perception. Did you spot the gorilla walking past the basketball players the first time you saw Daniel Simons's famous selective attention test on YouTube?[7] What we perceive is not always what's right in front of us.

Hallucinations, then, are not necessarily evidence of mental illness at all. But are they also compatible with being normal? A decade or so back, I took part in a pilot training course to help people understand and support mental health in the workplace. One session I remember particularly clearly. It started with the leaders encouraging us, in pairs, to share everyday experiences that might help us to appreciate some of the extremes of psychosis. 'How about', I suggested to my partner, a middle-aged security guard who seemed rather anxious just to be in the room, 'when you think you hear someone calling your name but you turn round and there's no one there?' The man looked immediately horrified. 'But isn't that ... normal?'

he stammered. Well, yes. That was the whole point of the exercise, after all.

This man's fear that he might be judged abnormal reflects the widespread assumption today that seeing or hearing things that aren't objectively real is worryingly pathological. 'It is generally agreed', wrote clinical psychologist Mary Boyle in the late twentieth century, 'that, while reactions differ across social groups, modern Western societies are particularly hostile' to hallucinations.[8]

In certain religious sects, in contrast, mystical experiences may be sought out through fasting, sleep deprivation, infliction of pain or social isolation. Hearing or seeing things that others don't has also not been consistently judged as mental illness across time. When historian Michael MacDonald explored the archive of early seventeenth-century astrological physician Richard Napier, he found that while many people visited Napier for help with mental distress or unorthodox behaviour, hallucinations were not commonly reported as a problem.[9] MacDonald concluded that, within the religious and cultural context of the time, these experiences were more readily understandable. Hearing the voice of God was a spiritual experience, while viewing supernatural beings or witnessing magical practices could be taken at face value at this time, even by a physician.

Joseph Kirk's vision of his maid in 1886 was one of many 'hallucinations of the sane' reported in a Census of Hallucinations compiled by the Society for Psychical Research (SPR). Founded in 1882, the SPR aimed to scientifically investigate paranormal phenomena, from ghostly visitations to seances and telepathy. While some members of the SPR considered the late Victorian vogue for the supernatural to be an immense hoax, others were open to the suggestion that 'wider laws or a larger circle of phenomena ... may exist, and may still be discovered', as psychiatrist and SPR sympathiser Daniel Hack Tuke poetically put it.[10] 'Membership of this Society', the SPR constitution read, 'does not imply the acceptance of any particular explanation of the phenomena investigated, nor any belief as to the operation, in the physical world, of forces other than those recognised by physical science.'[11] The truth might be out there ... but equally it might not be. Unlike Fox Mulder in *The X-Files*, the SPR were carefully hedging their bets.

Their census began in 1889 and was completed in 1892. 'Have you ever,' the census survey asked, 'when believing yourself to be completely awake, had a vivid impression of seeing, or being touched by a living being, or inanimate object, or of hearing a voice; which impression, so far as you could discover, was not due to any external physical cause?' Out of the 17,000 respondents, 2,272 replied that they had: approximately 13 per cent of the total.[12] Of course, one can easily take issue with the SPR's sampling techniques – as in many Victorian surveys, dissemination relied heavily on the friendship networks of the researchers – or their aim to use the survey to explore the mechanism of telepathic communication. The census was, however, one of the first statistical studies of visual and auditory hallucinations.

The Census of Hallucinations concluded that, while it was not an everyday experience for most people, seeing things and hearing voices was also not proof of abnormality.

The assumption that hallucinations were pathological, remarked author Edmund Gurney, had retarded efforts to understand them. There is a 'certain vague prejudice', Gurney wrote, 'in the minds of persons who have never met with an instance of hallucination of any sort. Such persons can often hardly bring themselves to conceive that a sane, healthy, waking mind can really get momentarily off the rails, and can feign voices where there is silence, and figures where there is vacancy.'[13]

Twentieth-century studies have found similar results to the SPR, reporting that between 10 and 50 per cent of people experience hallucinations of sight or hearing at some point in their lives.[14] These experiences are not, of course, always benign. Yet neither are they necessarily distressing or unpleasant, even in today's world. It's when people struggle to incorporate them into their lives or explain them to others that they often become a problem.

Eleanor Longden, of the Hearing Voices Network, or HVN, speaks of this in her 2013 TED talk and book on her experience of psychiatric care in the early 2000s. Longden was a student when she began to hear voices narrating her every move. At first it didn't really trouble her; it was only after a friend and then a doctor told Longden she was seriously unwell that her life began to unravel. The voices became so bad that Longden's parents had to stop her drilling a hole in her head to try to get them out, and she was diagnosed with schizophrenia. Nothing helped, until a psychiatrist finally encouraged her to look for meaning in the voices and respond to them: finally, things began to improve. In 2013, Eleanor Longden still heard voices, but had learned how to listen to and manage them.

Today, groups like HVN advocate for those who hear voices and see visions.[15] 'Despite being relatively common,' their website states, 'many people who hear voices, see visions or have similar experiences feel alone. Fear of prejudice, discrimination, and being dismissed as "crazy" can keep people silent.' Yet 'the majority of people who hear voices are not diagnosed with any illness at all. Some find voices and visions an important part of their life.'[16]

Modern medicine has not done a great deal to enhance our understanding of hallucinations, even if peer support networks like HVN have done a lot to advocate for those who experience them. Voice-hearing may, after all, be compatible with so-called normal life. It may also be a daily struggle to manage, coping with the reactions of others alongside the intrusive and often painful content of hallucinations. I once sat in on an HVN support group in South London as participants discussed their ideas and thoughts. One woman shared a wistful desire to go into a coffee shop and be treated as normal, not marked out as different by her behaviour. Others talked of their coping strategies – music, meditation or distraction – a necessary aspect of life given that, despite heavy medication, everyone in the group continued to hear voices, especially in times of stress. 'What's the one thing you'd most like people to understand about voice-hearing?' the facilitator asked the group. A quiet young man, who had barely spoken during the session, immediately opened his mouth. 'That it's not just the case that you take a drug and everything's normal.'

THE GREAT ABNORMALS

Over the course of the nineteenth and early twentieth centuries, the line between sane and insane became
increasingly blurred. This was not only because less common experiences like hearing voices and seeing visions
were reinterpreted; so, too, were more widespread features of mental life, from emotional distress to worry and
anxiety. While early nineteenth-century psychiatrists had
assumed that the majority of people were, to all intents
and purposes, mentally normal, their later counterparts
set greater store in a spectrum of mental health. This not
only reframed the way ordinary people viewed their minds,
but greatly expanded the number of people considered
not quite normal. And when Freud finally declared that
we were *all* neurotics, the normal mind became quite the
conundrum. It was usual, but unhealthy, to be neurotic. Yet
it was unusual – or well-nigh impossible! – to be entirely
healthy. So, which of these was actually 'normal'?

'We may compare the course of mental evolution to
a broad roadway,' explained the wonderfully named psychiatrist Theophilus Bulkeley Hyslop (T.B. to his friends)
in a popular book called *The Borderland* in 1925. On the
narrow footpath march the sane – 'comparatively safe'
unless accident or injury should strike. In the gutter are
those who have fallen from the wayside, 'the criminal, the
drunkard and the dement'. In between lies the vast road of
life, through which the majority pass in their struggle for
survival, a tumultuous throng of noise and nerves. Labelled
either as eccentrics or visionaries, the bulk of humanity are
'erratic, erotic, and unstable', said Hyslop, travelling at a

pace that makes them unsafe to themselves and others.[17] In statistical terms this vast multitude that so threatened Hyslop were the normal or average of the population; in medical terms, they were all neurotic.

Theo Hyslop – as T.B. was known professionally – is an interesting character through which to trace the emerging concern with neurosis. By the time he wrote *The Borderland* Hyslop was in his sixties and had been in private practice for over a decade. His later publications point to an opinionated, contradictory and at times old-fashioned individual who, despite living in London, blamed the noise and stress of city life for physical and mental degeneration (or 'brain fag', as he called it).[18]

Hyslop's professional life and career spanned the heyday of the 'borderland'. Born in 1863, the young Theo was literally brought up in an asylum; when he was two years old, his father William purchased Stretton House in Shropshire. As in most institutions, the superintendent's family lived on-site. This inspired Theo to train as a doctor, later specialising in psychiatry and working at Bethlem for over two decades, until he moved into private practice in 1910. He was also a keen artist, writer and musician, and a member of a range of social and political groups.

When Hyslop is noticed at all by today's writers, it's usually as a misanthropic advocate of eugenics, who despised his patients and railed against artistic modernism as the madness of modernity (he really wasn't keen on Roger Fry and the Bloomsbury Group).[19] The reality is more complicated. Indeed, some of Hyslop's closest friends at Bethlem seem to have been his patients. In the preface to his textbook, *Mental Physiology*, Hyslop thanked three people: one was Maurice Craig, a junior colleague; the other two were patients, Walter Abraham Haigh and Henry Francis Harding. Indeed, Hyslop's frustration at the neurotic multitude outside the asylum seems to have emerged from a romanticised view of madness itself. In his 'sort of novel' – as a colleague damningly described it – *Laputa, Revisited by Gulliver Redivivus in 1905,* the inhabitants of the Laputan asylum share a 'spirit of truth and integrity', and beyond some 'eccentricities of conduct there was little to distinguish them from the so-called sane'.[20]

The same year as *The Borderland* was published, Hyslop also penned a book with the revealing title *The Great Abnormals*. This rather confused volume of historical and philosophical ramblings about tyrants and despots, visionaries, witchcraft, superstition and men of genius was, Hyslop declared, a 'plea for the greater spirit of tolerance'. He pointed out that while there are 'those who do not conform to our own self-opinionated standards of mentality' nonetheless some of the 'individuals whose "abnormalities" [are] about to be described have been among "the great ones of the earth"'.[21] If greater tolerance was practised, Hyslop had no doubt, men of genius would no longer have to seek 'havens of refuge' (by which he meant asylums) to hide their 'eccentric, unconventional, or abnormal' behaviour.[22] They probably still shouldn't have children, though, he warned.

Hyslop may have had his friend Walter in mind here. Walter Haigh had been in and out of Bethlem since 1882, when he was first admitted at the age of twenty-seven. He was university-educated, worked as a teacher, and wrote and performed music in his spare time. Haigh also suffered from hallucinations and delusions, including a paranoia so intense that, even when he was given a free pass to go outside the hospital, he never used it. After Hyslop arrived at Bethlem in 1888, the two musicians seem to have become close. Haigh stayed in regular contact with Hyslop by letter, discussing work and home as well as his ongoing symptoms. Walter Haigh almost always put the words 'sane' and 'insane' in quotation marks, suggesting that sanity and insanity were relative terms. Hyslop later started to refer to 'so-called insanity' in his textbooks, perhaps inspired by his friend.[23]

Theo Hyslop's hostility towards the borderland of neurotic persons was in part a loyalty to those who had fallen by the wayside. Hyslop – as a presumably sane individual – had more in common with the 'mad' Walter Haigh than he did with the unhealthy, neurotic multitude: or so he thought. When the psychiatrist died in 1933, a former colleague noted that Hyslop's later years were 'saddened by something in the nature of a neurosis', an anxiety state which emerged during the air raids of the First World War and later became manifest as a tic of shoulders and face. T.B. was, after all, neurotic and therefore quite normal.

By the 1880s, most psychiatrists took it as read that sanity and insanity were different in degree rather than in kind. While they remained polar opposites, the two were now separated by a very large group of individuals 'saturated with the seeds of nervous disorders'.[24] But how were doctors to recognise the inhabitants of this borderland? To put it simply, they were all 'classes of person' who neglected the 'simpler conventions of society', from the sexually deranged to social misfits, hypochondriacs and self-mutilators.[25] Their neurosis was defined against the expectations of their families, peers and social leaders. Their behaviour might be distressing or harmful to others, or it might simply be inconvenient. Either way, the definition of abnormality consisted largely of unconventional acts. And this behaviour was newly interpreted as in need of medical attention.

Of course, many Victorian conventions seem highly unusual to us now, making clear just how closely definitions of the abnormal mind relied on social expectation (and still do). In October 1895, the young socialist Edith Lanchester – mother of *Bride of Frankenstein* actress Elsa Lanchester – announced to her wealthy father that she intended to move in with her working-class lover. Her father was horrified and immediately called for elderly psychiatrist George Fielding Blandford, who certified twenty-four-year-old Edith as insane. Blandford deemed the young woman's decision to live unmarried with a man – from a different social class, no less! – to be 'social suicide'. Her actions not only flouted convention but promised to do her status considerable future harm. Edith was taken to Roehampton Asylum, 'not without some struggling and force', although she was almost as quickly discharged by two Commissioners in Lunacy (the state asylum inspectors) who overruled Blandford's certificate.[26]

In 1896, the *Journal of Mental Science* published a carefully worded defence of Blandford, implying that while a decision to flout normal convention should not automatically result in a verdict of insanity, it was nonetheless possible that Edith Lanchester's actions had been the result of madness.[27] The court disagreed, and Lanchester was confirmed sane. However, this case clearly shows how, over the last hundred years and more, people ruled as insane have often come to the attention of authorities because of their unconventional behaviour. While those with wealth and power might be able to fight the judgements made about them, others could not. Those most likely to experience the negative effects of diagnosis were the 'marginalised, the vulnerable, and the dispossessed of twentieth-century society': unmarried women, Black people, older people, political dissidents, conscientious objectors, LGBTQ people, homeless people and more.[28] In 1851, American physician Samuel Cartwright even invented a new disease – drapetomania – with which he diagnosed runaway slaves. Running away was not, according to Cartwright, a rational response to the brutal treatment and lack of freedom experienced by slaves in the US but was 'as much a disease of the mind as any other species of mental alienation'.[29]

Sanity could be a powerful tool of social and legal control. Cartwright sought to 'normalise' the slaves he treated by telling their owners to ensure any Black person was kept 'in the position that we learn from the Scriptures he was intended to occupy, that is, the position of submission', an overtly racist perspective on medical control.[30] In the same century, middle-class women diagnosed with hysteria, like novelist Charlotte Perkins Gilman, were subjected to 'rest cures' that prescribed bed rest, seclusion, electricity, massage and over-feeding.[31] This too was designed to keep them in a position of submission – though with considerably less physical brutally, of course. Denied access to her books and work, Gilman wrote damningly

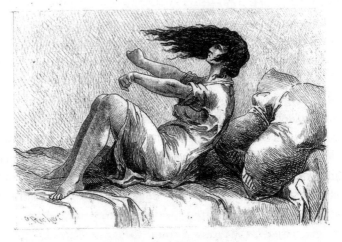

Fig. 1.　　　　Phase des grands mouvements

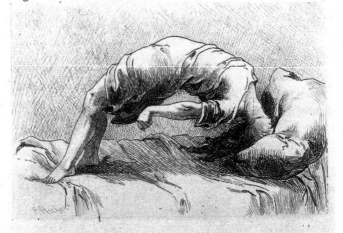

Fig. 2.　　　　Phase des contorsions
(Arc de cercle.)

Two of neurologist Jean-Martin Charcot's phases of hysteria, 1881. Charcot famously claimed there was a set pattern to hysteria, though this wasn't apparent outside his hospital.

of the mind-numbing boredom of her experience in *The Yellow Wallpaper*, published in 1892.

Hysteria was, as historian Elaine Showalter put it, the quintessential 'female malady'.[32] Although men *were* also diagnosed with hysteria, the very term – from the Greek for 'womb' – emphasised its feminine origin. Men were more often diagnosed with neurasthenia, the 'disease of civilization' introduced by the American neurologist George Miller Beard in 1869. Neurasthenia, as the beardless Beard described it, was a form of nervous exhaustion. Modern life was undoubtedly to blame, for it demanded the constant expenditure of mental energy, which exhausted the nerves. This, Beard said, caused headaches, joint pain, neuralgia, irritability, morbid fears, chills, tremors, sweating, sleeplessness and a whole host of other physical and mental symptoms. Luckily, it was also a marker of social status. Neurasthenia was a disease of wealth and education, most common in white Americans and found in 'nearly every brain-working household'.[33] (Working-class men or Black people who exhibited the same symptoms, he implied, were probably just lazy.)

Like neurasthenia, hysteria had a huge range of symptoms and was often a diagnosis of last resort when no physical explanation could be found – especially if the patient was young, female and unmarried. Hysteria might manifest as blindness, paralysis, spasms, fits, fainting, exhaustion, emotional outbursts and more. Unconventional behaviour might also be blamed for producing nervous symptoms in the first place. When Evelyn Jones was admitted to Bethlem Hospital in 1895, her illness was thought to stem from her reading of Darwin and other scientific books, as well as her very close relationship with a female friend.[34]

Marriage became a common recommendation to cure female nervous disorders. Alice Rose Morison, a twenty-five-year-old teacher from Harpenden, discovered this when she consulted eminent neurologist Victor Horsley in 1894. Alice had been sleepwalking for the past four years. This worried her because at times she went right out into the street, on one occasion walking all the way to her sister's lodgings. Sometimes she lit a fire or carried out other dangerous tasks. She also made a great deal of noise, banging at the door and hitting her head on the floor. Around Christmas 1893, Alice Morison started writing letters in her sleep, and the following summer began to go into trances during the day. Around this time, additional personalities emerged: Nocturna took over Alice's body at night, while a third mischievous state hid and stole things unknown to 'Morison', as she called her original self. In July 1894, when she went to see Dr Horsley, Alice found herself annoyed by his dismissive suggestion that 'rest and marriage' would cure her. She 'would not follow his advice', the determined young woman later told psychiatrists at Bethlem Hospital.[35]

Other women were pressed by family, friends and medical professionals into the conventional route of marriage and children. To behave normally was to be cured. In the 1880s and 1890s, many doctors thought marriage would 'cure nervous evils', even as others worried that this risked proliferating a nervous strain in the population, increasing the number of unstable people still further.[36] Andrew Wynter – the first cartographer of the borderlands – suggested that changes in the circumstances of women had caused a rise in alcoholism. The middle-class woman was imperfectly educated, separated from her husband by the new railway that allowed him to commute to work and gave all her housework to servants. In such a situation, Wynter wondered, how could one expect bored and isolated housewives to 'become sensible wives'?[37] If only women had enough housework to do, normality would be resumed.

It might not be hard to accept the idea that neuroses are shaped by the society around us. It is, however, equally easy to assume that there are some categories of mental illness that remain stable. Yet, no matter how damaging and distressing some experiences of mental ill health might be – to those going through them and others who care about them – they are rarely quite so alien from our own lives as we are led to believe. Nor do they colour every aspect of a person's existence. Normal behaviour – in any sense of the term – is certainly not incompatible with madness, just as abnormal behaviour and experiences are not incompatible with sanity. That's why the message that has stayed with me throughout my research are the wry words of Theo Hyslop in 1895. 'We must, as presumably sane individuals, be generous in the limits we assign to the interpretations which others give to their own experiences.'[38]

NEUROSIS IS THE NEW NORMAL

What is consciousness? Even today, the concept is 'notoriously ambiguous', according to one recent collection of philosophical essays on the subject.[39] By 'conscious', do we simply mean awake and aware? Do we have an inner self, that observes and interprets the world around us, or is the very idea of self a product of the narrative created by our conscious thought? If the former, then a split or multiple self seems abnormal; if the latter, multiple selves may be more understandable. In the age of hysteria, consciousness could be split, fractured or multiplied. It could be altered by hypnotism or trances. It had multiple levels: there was a subliminal consciousness, a subconscious or an unconscious. The experiences of Alice Morison and others like her brought into question the idea of a single, unified consciousness, which had previously seemed the very definition of a 'normal' mind.

Alice Morison was not the first case of 'double consciousness' recorded.[40] In France, teenage seamstress Félida X began to see a doctor in 1858 after regular lapses into a second state, whose actions and words were immediately forgotten on returning to her 'normal state' (as her doctor called it). Over time, the second state became the usual one, and Félida's original state disappeared.[41] Charcot's student Pierre Janet hypnotised one of his patients to produce similar results. Léonie B., a middle-aged peasant woman, could be mesmerised into a livelier personality she called Léontine. Later, Janet managed to produce a 'Léonie 3' (or Léonore), who appeared to be a separate entity once again.[42] These multiple personalities, suggested psychologists and philosophers across Europe, Britain and the US, might help us better understand not only hysteria, but normal consciousness itself.

Except it didn't happen quite like that. By the early twentieth century, hypnotism and psychical research were seeming increasingly dubious. By the time SPR founder Frederic Myers's *Human Personality and Its Survival of Bodily Death* was published – posthumously, of course – in 1903, the connections between spiritualism and psychology were beginning to fracture. This wasn't the end of the study of the 'supernormal' (as Myers himself dubbed it), but the normal mind was beginning to take a new direction. And one reason for this was very simple: Sigmund Freud was rubbish at hypnosis.

Instead of hypnotising his patients, as Janet and others had done, the young Viennese neurologist sat behind them and interpreted their speech instead. This was certainly a major difference between Freud's approach and that of his mentor, Josef Breuer, who employed cathartic hypnosis with his patients. It was, nonetheless, Breuer's 'hysterical' patient who became famous for her role in the foundation of psychoanalysis. Fräulein 'Anna O.' was later identified as Bertha Pappenheim, an Austrian feminist and later the founder of the Jewish Women's Association. Pappenheim was twenty-two years old when Breuer first treated her in 1881, and 'bubbling over with intellectual vitality', despite leading an 'extremely monotonous existence in her puritanically-minded family'.[43] It was the mundanity of normal life for middle-class European women, Breuer and Freud concluded, which had resulted in the development of Bertha Pappenheim's abnormal state of mind.

Pappenheim's first symptom was 'systematic day-dreaming', quickly followed by signs more noticeable to her family: a squint, severe disturbances of vision, paralysis and contracture of the limbs and persistent somnambulism (sleepwalking). Between 11 December 1880 and 1 April

1881, she was bed bound. In April, Pappenheim began her treatment with Breuer. Her symptoms were serious, and 'it was only for a short time during the day that she was to any degree normal'.[44] During the therapy, she and Breuer discussed the appearance of each symptom, relating them to occurrences in her earlier life, such as the illness and death of her father. The doctor found, to his surprise, that 'each symptom disappeared after she had described its first occurrence' under hypnosis.[45] Historians have viewed Anna O.'s treatment rather differently. The process of recollection occurred late in Breuer's treatment of Pappenheim and does not seem to have led to the long-term cure that Breuer implied it did.[46]

Breuer called his treatment of Anna O. a 'talking cure': a phrase which would become indelibly associated with his protégé. Today, it is often assumed that Freud was the first person to use psychological methods in the treatment of mental illness. Many people also regard Freud as the first physician to view madness on a continuum, from psychosis to neurosis to normal health. This, as we have already seen, is simply not true. Freud was not even the first or only person to adopt psychotherapy, a word already in occasional use to imply direct or indirect suggestion in mental health care.[47] Yet, although he ultimately became as much a personality cult as a scientist, Freud did emphasise several things that became important in the history of the normal mind: the role of childhood development, and the expansion of the abnormal beyond even the borderlands.

For Freud, we are *all* neurotic, right down to the very fringes of the normal curve. As he wrote in his famous break-up letter to his own protégé Carl Jung in 1913, 'It is

Advert for Baldwin's Nervous Pills, one of many patent remedies that claimed to cure hysteria and other 'nerve pains and diseases', c.1900.

a convention among us analysts that none of us need feel ashamed of his own bit of neurosis.' Jung, Freud claimed, was a man who 'while behaving abnormally keeps shouting that he is normal'. This indicated a lack of insight, which could not be tolerated. 'I propose that we abandon our personal relations entirely,' Freud angrily concluded.[48] It was not necessarily a problem not to be normal, so long as one was aware of it.

After Freud, the normal mind vanished from the realms of possibility. This helpfully served to increase the popularity of psychoanalysis until, long after Freud died in 1939, anybody who was anybody was expected to be seeing a therapist, especially in the US. 'Neurotic' became a figure of speech rather than a diagnosis: a flippant description of behaviour or a self-deprecating comment. Yet the idea of neurosis also shaped our lives, heightening late twentieth-century fears about the normality of our minds. What did a fear of spiders or open spaces say about us, we began to wonder? Did unusual behaviour in adult life imply some deep, dark secret of our childhoods? No longer a distant threat, as it had been for the very early Victorians, the abnormal was perpetually there, a shadow behind our every act, threatening daily to overwhelm us.

WHAT IS A NORMAL MIND?

Have *you* ever worried that you might be going mad? When I took a class in the history of madness in my late twenties, this was one of the first things the tutor asked us. A good three-quarters of the class immediately admitted they had.

Those who did not felt awkward, singled out – perhaps, like Carl Jung, fearing a lack of insight. 'I've never worried about going mad!' one of the group protested, anxiously gazing round at the forest of hands. 'Does that mean I'm *not* normal?' Psychiatrists in the late nineteenth and early twentieth centuries would probably have thought her one of the lucky few with good mental health. Her words, however, reflect the growing assumption post-Freud that those who have never questioned their sanity are simply deluded.

Despite these fears, many of us continue to try to retain a boundary between our everyday fears and what we consider outright insanity. While late Victorian psychiatrists thought most people were mentally abnormal and Freud contended that pretty much everyone was, the recent statistic is more comforting: 'one in four'. Mental health charities and anti-stigma campaigns have been telling us since the early 2000s that one in four of us will experience a mental health problem at some point in our lives. This is far less widespread than Freud assumed, even if it nonetheless indicates that mental distress is a relatively common occurrence.

But where does this statistic come from? The figure appeared at the start of the twenty-first century, in a World Health Organization report which made this striking claim: 'During their entire lifetime, more than 25 per cent of individuals develop one or more mental or behavioural disorders.'[49] When a psychiatrist and a neuroscientist – Stephen Ginn and Jamie Horder – followed the references from this paper, they discovered that the mysterious figure had appeared out of thin air.[50] None of the three papers the study cited actually made this claim at all: in fact, two gave a considerably higher figure for lifetime prevalence of mental disorders.

The only study Ginn and Horder could find that gave a figure of approximately a quarter was the annual Adult Psychiatric Morbidity Survey (APMS). This found that 23 per cent of people in the UK had experienced a mental health problem in the past week alone. Any lifetime figure extrapolated from this would, of course, be significantly higher than 23 per cent. Ginn and Horder also found significant differences between studies as to what constituted mental illness. Some disorders that *are* listed in the DSM – including 'male erectile disorder' and 'nicotine dependence' (I kid you not) – were not included in most surveys. The addition of ADHD (attention deficit hyperactivity disorder) to a 2010 study led to a huge increase in the prevalence of mental health problems. Ginn and Horder concluded that one in four had proven popular not because it was supported by evidence but simply because it was 'not too big, not too small'.[51] It makes our distressing experiences seem acceptable, but also gives us hope that they will end. Lifetime estimates of mental illness across a range of countries, however, have suggested a figure closer to half.[52] In other words, mental illness is actually pretty normal, statistically speaking.

The journey we have taken into the ever-expanding borderlands of insanity, however, shows how drastically the definition of what's normal or abnormal in mind has shifted, both medically and socially. While Victorian psychiatrists recognised that normality was shaped by social convention, they nonetheless assumed that many people *were* entirely sane. Following conventional pursuits was recommended as a cure for those who didn't fit into the narrow boundaries imposed on them: hysterical girls should get married; alcoholic housewives just needed to do a bit more cleaning and childcare. Today, we might put our faith in a chemical or neurological model of emotion and behaviour that is not always conducive to our well-being. Sometimes this blinds us to the social expectations that continue to shape our attitudes to normal and abnormal behaviour. Of course, in our darkest moments, medicine may support or sustain us. But it can also trap us into a narrow interpretation of experiences.

Let's close with one last attempt to define the normal mind, at the University of Michigan Hospital in 1967. This study hoped to generate a definition of normal that could be applied in a more coherent way to mental health. A group of trainee psychiatrists and a group of people diagnosed with schizophrenia were given the same test. How, participants were asked, would a 'typical normal person' react in any given situation? In one example, subjects were asked to consider the reaction of this 'typical normal person' if his boss called him a 'stupid idiot' in front of colleagues. The responses of psychiatrists alone ranged from 'annoyed but decides to forget the whole thing' to 'much anger – quits his job'. While the sample was very small, the researchers found this variation significant.[53] In other words, normal people had wildly different opinions about what constituted normal behaviour.

The 'state hospital schizophrenics' – a horribly reductive description – showed even greater variation than the psychiatrists. This group veered towards the milder end of the scale. While no trainee psychiatrist thought a normal person would not care at all when called a 'stupid idiot', 10 per cent of people diagnosed with schizophrenia plumped for this option. Thirty-one per cent of psychiatric patients also plumped for a mild response ('annoyed but decides to forget'), while only 8 per cent of trainees did the same.

What are we to make of these differences? Does it mean that some people with a diagnosis of schizophrenia are less bothered by the actions of other people than the supposedly 'normal' psychiatrists? Or was it perhaps that these hospital patients had much more to gain or lose from the definition of what's normal? Their responses to the test were in all likelihood shaped by the centrality of this notion to their experiences of being diagnosed as mentally ill. As a study of mental hospital life a decade earlier had pointed out, the 'concept of "normal", and the implied promise of everything that a patient may imagine as included in it, is the dominant conscious organizing factor in everything a patient does in the hospital'.[54] To be recognised as normal by others might lead to earlier discharge; to behave in a range of sanctioned 'abnormal' ways could result in harsh treatments or the withdrawal of privileges.

This highly loaded notion of normalcy remains significant in mental health care today. There is often little space for cultural difference. As in the University of Michigan survey, definitions of normal behaviour tend to privilege the lifestyles and experiences of well-paid professionals over those of their patients. Just as male psychiatrists in the late nineteenth century made assumptions about the proper social behaviour of women, so too an upper-middle-class psychiatrist today brings their own assumptions and biases. A trip to the supermarket seems like an easy thing to do when you have a car and a credit card and a childminder and a tendency to forget that other people don't have these things. When ideas of normalcy are based – as they so often are – on a particular middle-class life-style, it becomes even harder for those outside this realm to conform. And yet not conforming is nonetheless regarded as a sign of illness.

These notions of normalcy are drawn along lines of age, gender, class and race. When I was in my early twenties and struggling with severe depression, one night out in the pub with friends suddenly erupted into crisis. I eventually ended up in A&E, but not before the neighbours called the police as my flatmate and boyfriend fought in the hallway. The cops arrived to find me covered in blood. 'Who did this to you?' they asked me again and again, pointing at the wounds on my arm. 'Was it your boyfriend?' Confronted by a distressed and injured young woman in an East London council block, the police assumed domestic violence. When I eventually managed to tell them I'd harmed myself, they left: job done.

But what if I'd been a Black man, in the same situa-tion? Would the police have treated me in the same way, or would they have interpreted my distress as a threat? The Count Me In census of 2010 found that admission rates for mental health inpatients across 238 NHS and private hos-pitals in the UK were two to six times higher than average for some groups of Black people. This was largely due to a high rate of hospitalisation among those of Black African and Caribbean descent, who were also more likely to be admitted involuntarily, often through the criminal justice system.[55] Psychiatrists argued whether or not this proved that psychiatry was institutionally racist. Wasn't it a good thing, one respondent insisted, that so many people had been handed over by the police and the courts to receive the treatment they needed?[56] But what did their apprehension by the police in the first place say about the different ways behaviour is interpreted and understood, or the (often violent) way some people are handled by the authorities? These inequalities, as we have seen, are not just part of psychiatry but embedded throughout the history of science and medicine, of law, policing and psychology. It's hard to see how psychiatry could escape being institutionally racist when the rest of society is.

4

IS MY SEX LIFE NORMAL?

Like most young Londoners in the early 2000s, I lived in a shared house throughout my twenties. Sex was a frequent topic of conversation, often through in-jokes and coded language. We had a wall of 'husbands' (celebrities we fancied) covering up a huge garish mirror in the living room of our rented house. 'Just making the tea' became a private joke, the phrase sparking knowing laughter since no one outside our group would understand the sexual connotations. We giggled about squeaky beds, 'hairy naked guy' who could never remember whose room he was sharing after an early-morning toilet trip, or the strange things new partners said or did at orgasm. We wrote and shared a hell of a lot of explicit fanfic.

Despite our giggles and anxieties, we all thought of ourselves as more or less normal. Our ideas of shared living were based on the 1990s TV shows we'd grown up with – *Friends* or *This Life* or perhaps even *Buffy the Vampire Slayer* – in which (almost) everyone was young, attractive, white and heterosexual. *Buffy the Vampire Slayer* was especially hung up on sex. When Buffy loses her virginity, her boyfriend quite literally becomes evil and tries to destroy the world. And there's one moment in the *Buffy* musical – which we sang along to over and over – that highlights the insidious nature of the norms that thread through many of these shows. Girlfriends Willow and Tara make an excuse to leave their friends and go home, ostensibly to have sex. When Buffy's teenage sister Dawn calls this 'kinda romantic', Buffy and her friend Xander immediately jump in to contradict, with a horrified, 'No it's not!' Why not? Is the implication that lesbian sex isn't romantic? Or that Dawn, as a teenager, needs to be protected from sex entirely?

To better understand the norms around consensual sex, we need to delve into their history.* One 1940s study suggested that everyone held a highly personal definition of sexual normalcy, based on vague notions about how other people behave. It found two main ways in which people judge abnormal sexual behaviour: the nature of sex acts themselves and the frequency of sexual activity. Yet the way in which individuals came to their conclusions about what act or frequency was normal was complex and confusing, based on a 'conglomeration of ill-sorted ideas, half absorbed, half understood, often half-rejected' from sources as diverse as the movie screen, the psychiatrist's couch, the pulpit, the doctor's surgery, the street corner and the birth control clinic.[1] 'Ideas of normality to some extent

---

* While rape, assault and paedophilia may occur with a frequency that speaks volumes about the power relations and conventions within our society and can even become disturbingly 'normalised' in certain social contexts, I will be focusing in this chapter on consensual sex. To read more on the history of rape, see Joanna Bourke, *Rape: A History from 1860 to the Present* (London: Virago, 2007).

govern ideas of morality,' the report went on. However, 'uncertainty as to what other people do may make it more difficult than ever for the man in the street to decide just what is normal and what is not'.

This idea of a personal notion of normality fails, however, to acknowledge how law, medicine and social expectation have impacted significantly on the way people expect others to live their lives. Between 1885 and 1967, any sex act between two men was against the law in the United Kingdom, as in many other countries. In some parts of the world people continue to be imprisoned or even put to death for having intimate relations with someone of the same gender. Women – and women of colour especially – have suffered social and legal repercussions from sex outside marriage and having illegitimate children and, in some countries, adultery remains a criminal offence. The history of sexuality, then, is also a history of legal and medical control, of the coercion of certain people by others, and of the exclusion and oppression of those deemed to be sexually 'different'.

The way coercion and control are bound up in the history of sex frustrates the modern Western assumption that consensual sex is something that all healthy people ought to enjoy. And sex remains complicated. Many of us are still ashamed or embarrassed by our sexual interests, or uncertain about the reactions of others. I remember being mortified when a new boyfriend visited my house for the first time only to look rather daunted by *The Encyclopedia of Unusual Sex Practices* sitting on my bedside table. 'It's for, er, research,' I stammered. He nervously changed the subject. Top-shelf magazines retain a furtive, embarrassing aura, and piles of unrelated serious books continue to mask the windows of Soho dirty bookshops. And sex sells newspapers, films and books too, of course. Would it have captured the ears of the nation in the same way if, in 2015, it had been any other part of his anatomy that then Prime Minister David Cameron allegedly put into a dead pig's mouth while at college?

We may think of sex as something sordid, secret and hidden, even as we consider it a normal part of our everyday lives. After all, when sex still takes place largely behind closed doors, how *can* we ever really know if our sex lives are normal?

THE HEINOUS SIN OF SELF-POLLUTION

Louis was a watchmaker in the Swiss city of Lausanne.* Until the age of seventeen, some time in the 1750s, he had been happy and energetic in his work and kept good health. At this tender age, young Louis became addicted to the dreaded habit of masturbation: once, twice, even three times a day! Before the end of the year, the young man began to feel weak and suffered a host of horrifying symptoms, forcing him to give up work and confining him to his bed. The physician Samuel-Auguste Tissot found the teenager 'more like a corpse than a living being', his body 'dry, emaciated, pale, dirty, exhaling a disagreeable odor, and almost motionless'. Not only this, but the young man

---

* 'Louis' is known simply as 'L.D.' in the treatise. I have taken the liberty of christening him with a common French name for ease of reading, given that he lived in a French-speaking region of Switzerland.

foamed at the mouth, a 'pale bloody discharge' ran from his nose, his bowels were incontinent and 'there was a constant discharge of seminal fluid'. Louis had no memory and could no longer read. Masturbation, Tissot warned, had sunk the youth 'far beneath the brute' and, despite the doctor's prescription of tonics, the young man died a few weeks later.[2]

For most of us today, masturbation probably wouldn't be the first 'abnormal' sex act to spring to mind. Yet even though it is now widely assumed to be a normal healthy behaviour, it retains a certain taboo, showing how complex our attitudes to sex remain. I remember giving a museum tour for A-level students a few years back. One of them innocently asked me what a couple of objects in the display case were – a Victorian anti-masturbation device alongside some Japanese sex aids. When I started to explain, the entire mixed-sex group blushed furiously, giggling every time I said the word 'masturbation'.

I would probably have been embarrassed, too, at their age. While teen magazines in the 1990s highly recommended masturbation as a way of understanding your own body, it remained something private, that you were supposed to work out for yourself and never on any account discuss with others. I remember assuming that touching yourself was a bit dirty, even though I can't recall anyone specifically telling me this. Indeed, as recently as 1994, when US Surgeon General Joycelyn Elders – the first African American to hold the post – suggested that masturbation should be taught to young people, she lost the support of Bill Clinton's White House and was later forced to resign.

What on earth made masturbation seem so morally

dubious that President Clinton, who would soon be embroiled in his own sex scandal with intern Monica Lewinsky, couldn't allow it to be spoken of openly? For over two centuries, masturbation was thought abnormal in every possible way: morally and medically; on social and religious grounds. It was the sex act that caused the *most* concern – and often the most revulsion – throughout much of this period. Euphemisms were evocative of these public warnings: self-pollution, self-abuse, the solitary vice. The case of Louis the watchmaker appeared in Tissot's *Diseases Caused by Masturbation*, first published in French in 1760. This was not long after masturbation became a topic of specifically medical concern; previously it had been only a vaguely unpleasant vice.[3] In London in 1712, an anonymous doctor published the panic-inducing title *Onania: or, the Heinous Sin of Self-Pollution and All Its Frightful Consequences (in Both Sexes) Considered with Spiritual and Physical Advice to Those Who Have already Injured Themselves by this Abominable Practice.*[4]

Luckily, *Onania* reassured its readers, there was a simple cure for the medical effects of self-pollution. Anyone affected by discharges, infertility, impotence, or the countless other self-injuries associated with masturbation had only to look for the discreet Sign of the Bell in Paternoster Row, coincidentally the location of *Onania*'s publisher. Here they could purchase a marvellous 'Strengthening Tincture' and a 'Prolifick Powder' to restore them to health and vitality: and, if they were very worried, a Decoction and Injection to help the first two remedies along.[5] Essentially, *Onania* was a very lengthy advert.

Nonetheless, *Onania* sparked a masturbation panic that enveloped medicine throughout the eighteenth and nineteenth centuries. Historian Thomas Laqueur suggests that it struck a nerve in an era when morality was explicitly associated with self-governance for the first time.[6] Since self-control was now an individual matter, no longer shaped by an external relationship with God, self-love came to represent the threat the selfish and self-indulgent individual might hold for society.

ONANIA: OR, THE HEINOUS SIN OF *Self-Pollution*, AND ALL ITS FRIGHTFUL CONSEQUENCES (in Both Sexes) CONSIDERED,

With Spiritual and Physical ADVICE to those who have already injured themselves by this abominable Practice.

The frontispiece to the eighteenth edition of *Onania* (1756), the book that sparked a two-century masturbation panic.

The threat of solitary selfishness marked medical texts through the nineteenth century. And, where *Onania* had promised a quick cure, the Victorians worried that masturbation would cause long-term damage to the individual and society, to bodies and minds. Asylum superintendent Robert P. Ritchie claimed in 1861 that a remarkable 119 cases of insanity in his institution were caused by solitary sex, an early attempt to quantify masturbation's dreaded effects.[7] This formed 6.59 per cent of his male pauper patients and 12.52 per cent of male private patients: masturbation was a disease of the middle and upper classes, especially worrying to social order. 'Engaged in no social diversion, the patients of this group live alone in the midst of many,' Ritchie declared.

They did not talk with others, nor did they join in games or entertainments. They walked and sat alone. 'They seek no social joys, nor is the wish for fellowship evinced.' Solitary sex was very much a social, as well as a medical, problem.

By the last decade of the nineteenth century, things had calmed down a bit. Masturbation remained unpleasant, but doctors were coming to believe that it did not automatically result in wasting and death. If anything, though, this made them step up the incendiary language. Surgeon Sir James Paget described masturbation as 'so nasty a practice', 'a filthiness forbidden by God' and 'an unmanliness despised by men', that he wished he could claim occasional self-abuse to be more harmful to health than it actually was.[8] Asylum doctor David Yellowlees, meanwhile, called masturbation an 'incurable evil'. The masturbator shunned society. He had no intimate friends and did not dare to marry, nor even to 'look you in the face because he is haunted by the consciousness of a dirty secret which he must always conceal and always dreads that you may discover'.[9] Masturbation to the late Victorians was not just a sex act but affected the entire personality and behaviour of the masturbator. This shift, from abnormal act to abnormal person, is something we see time and again in the history of the normal.

Masturbation, many people agreed, turned the pleasant, normal youth into an abnormal, sullen fiend. It didn't matter that it was not dangerous to health and appeared to be widespread. Not that many tried to measure the prevalence of such a vile habit anyway. One rare man who did was Clement Dukes, the medical officer of Rugby School (though he doesn't tell us how). In 1884, Dukes suggested that a whopping 90–95 per cent of boarding school pupils masturbated: probably, he thought, because their usual bedtime fell a mere hour after a heavy supper.[10] Unable to sleep while they were still digesting, the boys turned instead to the solitary vice to send them off to dreamland.

The moral panic of the Victorian era focused on the male masturbator – even though, in 1712, *Onania* had claimed that masturbation was an equal problem for both sexes. As the century turned, gender equality began to return to the masturbation 'problem', largely thanks to British physician Havelock Ellis, who introduced the term 'auto-erotism' in 1898. Auto-erotism incorporated sexual daydreams and fantasies as well as physical manipulation, and women tended to admit to the former more often than the latter, said Ellis. He also argued that auto-erotism should not be viewed as either unnatural or pathological, since it was common to animals and 'the people of nearly every race of which we have any intimate knowledge'.[11] Even objects in the natural world seemed to indicate the normality of masturbation for women, like the banana, which 'appears to be marked out for the purpose by its size and shape'.[12] Everyday pastimes could cause sexual excitement: riding a horse or a bicycle, sitting on a train or even using a sewing machine. While some men suggested that this meant women's freedom should be curtailed, for Ellis it proved instead that sex, masturbation and fantasy were definitively normal, for men and women. What was *not* normal was the conflict between desire and convention.

Freud picked up on Ellis's ideas and made the idea of sexual conflict famous across the Western world. Unlike Ellis, Freud thought masturbation was only normal in certain circumstances. It was a stage in sexual development

– the 'lowest of the sexual strata' – that every child had to pass through.[13] Self-directed sex was natural in a young child, because their world revolved around their own physical needs. Normal sexual development, however, required a move beyond this to a sexual drive focused on others. Indeed, Freud even argued that masturbation caused harm if carried on at an age after which 'normal' sexual pursuits – in other words heterosexual penetrative intercourse – should have been adopted.[14]

It's hardly surprising, then, that ordinary people continued to worry about masturbation well into the twentieth century. After the publication of her bestseller *Married Love* in 1918, thousands of British people wrote to birth control advocate Marie Stopes to ask for advice, often revealing their anxieties about the physical, mental and marital effects of masturbation.* Men who wrote to Stopes during the Second World War, historian Lesley Hall discovered, were just as concerned about masturbation as those in 1918; the stigma hadn't faded.[15] 'As a result [of masturbation] I am very pale and awfully depressed,' wrote one young railway clerk mournfully in 1927; 'I cannot interest myself in anything, I am unfit for my work, sometimes I feel so depressed that I wish I was dead.'[16] While today we might attribute this young man's worries to poor mental health, he was certain that the headaches, aching eyes and bodily throbbing that accompanied his low mood were all due to his sexual habit. Indeed, pamphlets warning of 'Sexual Neurasthenia' and other medical perils brought on

---

* Like Havelock Ellis and many other writers on sex in the early twentieth century, Stopes was an outspoken supporter of eugenics, meaning her ideas must be viewed in the context of national sexual and social control.

by masturbation were still being advertised in newspapers and 'sex interest weeklies' after the Second World War.[17]

The medical profession continued to view masturbation as an unpleasant phase that young people ought to grow out of, after all. While Stopes replied sympathetically to the railway clerk, she nonetheless reminded him that it 'of course, is a habit which ought to be gradually checked and put a stop to'.[18] 'We have to restrain many impulses which are normal enough in themselves,' Dr Eustace Chesser counselled the teenage readers of *Grow Up – And Live* in 1949. 'Masturbation may be regarded as "normal", but it is wise and healthy to consider the reasons for doing your best to refrain.'[19] Masturbation, Chesser cautioned, might ruin a youth for a 'normal sex life' and reduce individual self-control, honour and decency – character advice that didn't differ much from Victorian medical writings. Masturbation might no longer be medically harmful, but it remained morally and socially problematic, ruining relationships and promoting anti-social behaviour.

Over two centuries the place of masturbation had shifted. From being just one among many sexual sins, it became the most dangerous of all, potentially even fatal. Self-love could waste the body and the mind, causing nervous illness while simultaneously producing a selfish, secretive, anti-social attitude. As psychologists and sexologists took up the topic in the early twentieth century, they clung to the latter belief even as they dismissed the former. If a healthy sex life meant marriage and heterosexual sex, then masturbation was its antithesis. Women who did not experience vaginal orgasm but could only be stimulated clitorally were, psychoanalysts decided, frigid.[20] That was no doubt why one 1940s woman was troubled by her occasional 'discharge of sexual energy' by masturbation and struggled to overcome a loathing of penetration.[21] Teenagers and adults alike continued to worry about whether or not masturbation was normal in the second half of the twentieth century. 'Did it make you go blind?' they wondered. 'Did it cause illness? Did it shrink the penis or enlarge the clitoris? Did it make you impotent, cause heart disease or make hair grow on the palms of the hands?' While the scientific answer to all of these questions was a resounding no, agony aunts in the 1970s and sex educators in the 1980s *still* found these worries to be widespread, a long legacy to earlier medical attitudes.[22]

SINS OF THE CITIES OF THE PLAIN

On 28 April 1870, two young ladies were arrested at the Strand Theatre in London. Mrs Fanny Graham and Miss Stella Boulton had somewhat bemused theatregoers with their behaviour. They appeared to be ladies of good social standing, yet their giggling, flirting and smoking suggested a lower social class, perhaps even that the women were prostitutes.[23] When the pair appeared at the Bow Street Magistrates' Court two days later, newspapers couldn't agree on how to describe them, other than by their clothing. The *Illustrated Police News* stated that Boulton, aged twenty-two, wore 'a cerise satin dress, with an "open square" body. The neck was hidden by the folds of a white lace scarf.' The newspaper made a point of adopting 'the pronoun used regarding the prisoner during the hearing of the case', noting that she wore a small signet ring and a golden wig, 'fashionably dressed in the Grecian style, with plaited chignon'.[24] *The Times* instead used male pronouns to describe the pair who had been charged with 'frequenting the Strand Theatre, with intent to commit felony', but showed a similar interest in their clothing. Boulton's co-defendant, the twenty-three-year-old law student who went by the name Fanny Graham, had on 'a dark green satin dress, low-necked, trimmed with black lace, of which material he also had a shawl round his shoulders. His hair was flaxen and in curls. He had on a pair of white kid gloves.'[25]

Today, we might want to label Fanny Graham and Stella Boulton – or Frederick William Park and Ernest Boulton as they were also known – as trans or gay, or perhaps more simply queer. They, in contrast, called themselves Mollies or Mary-Annes, a specific sub-culture that does not map neatly on to today's notions of sexual identity. Boulton and Park often dressed in women's clothing and used female pronouns, but also often did not. Indeed, when the pair first appeared in court, they wanted to change out of the dresses they were wearing when arrested, a request refused by the police.[26] Sometimes they

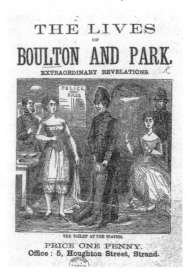

THE LIVES
OF
BOULTON AND PARK.
EXTRAORDINARY REVELATIONS.

THE TOILET AT THE STATION.

PRICE ONE PENNY.
Office : 5, Houghton Street, Strand.

Frontispiece of a 'penny dreadful' painting the Boulton and Park case as a lurid scandal, 1871.

played with the boundary between genders, wearing male clothing with make-up. They both used their given names as well as a variety of female names. At their trial, newspapers, witnesses and legal officials alike used both female and male pronouns to refer to Fanny and Stella, sometimes switching in the same sentence.[27] No one, it seemed, was quite sure where to place the pair.

So-called 'cross-dressing' was viewed as particularly subversive in the nineteenth century. As legal historian Judith Rowbotham notes, the practice was associated with political dissidents: Luddites, Irish insurgents and participants in the 'Rebecca Riots' of the 1830s and 1840s.[28] The police were also suspicious that men dressed as women might commit more mundane crimes while 'in disguise', such as theft and fraud: at first they suspected that Fanny and Stella were part of an elite pickpocketing gang.[29] What made the Boulton and Park trial significant is the fact that, unlike previous cases, it came to be about the sexual preferences and practices of those involved: Fanny, Stella and their six co-defendants.

The 1871 trial centred on the serious charge of conspiracy to commit sodomy, although the pair were ultimately found not guilty, in part thanks to conflicting medical evidence. Sodomy had been a capital offence until just a decade earlier, although the last execution took place in 1835. It was not synonymous with homosexuality: a heterosexual couple practising anal sex could also be charged. In the decade following Boulton and Park's trial, however, increasing legal, medical and public concern began to fall on the male homosexual as a particular kind of 'abnormal' sexual being. To put it simply, before the Boulton and Park trial there was – medically and legally at any rate – no such thing as a homosexual, only homosexual acts.

In the 1880s and 1890s, the idea that the homosexual was a type of person grew, often couched in gendered terms. Not that very many people used the term 'homosexual'. German lawyer Karl Heinrich Ulrichs called himself an 'Urning' or 'Uranian', a phrase drawn from classical mythology. The Urning was someone born with a male body and a female soul. This caused them to be sexually attracted to men and to view themselves as feminine in other ways. English writers Edward Carpenter and John Addington Symonds adopted the term and, although it was a more popular way of understanding same-sex relations in poetry and literature than in medicine, the notion of the feminised psyche took hold. In medical texts, same-sex encounters were defined in contrast to a 'norm' of opposite-sex practices: the clinical terms 'sexual inversion', 'sexual perversion' or 'antipathic sexual instinct' suggested a reversal or opposition. But of what exactly? The normal here was simply assumed.[30]

Yet this new medical view of pathological sexuality didn't stop Mary-Annes from congregating in Soho. Nor did it stop the cheerful debauchery of pornographic publications, like the entertaining *Sins of the Cities of the Plain*, published in 1881 – Oscar Wilde reportedly bought a copy in 1890.[31] The book was supposedly based on the recollections of a young prostitute, Jack Saul, and contains an amusing number of obsolete euphemisms, from gamahuching and copious spending to frigging and cockstands, which sounds more like a piece of furniture than an erection. The book also emphasised a link between homosexuality and gender inversion (Jack even, he claims, knew Fanny and Stella).[32]

Life was more difficult for many gay men whose memoirs survive, while queer people who did not identify as male are almost entirely absent from the record. John Addington Symonds worried with 'a passionate mixture of fascination and revulsion' about his 'fleeting encounters' with other men.[33] George Ives, founder of a secret club for gay men (the Order of Chaeronea) and self-described 'Sherlock Holmes of a 1000 little peculiarities', saw London as a city of danger and blackmail.[34] After all, across Europe, laws were being passed against 'gross indecency' between men 'in public or private', as Liberal MP Henry Labouchère's revision to Britain's 1885 Criminal Law Amendment Act put it.[35] It wasn't only sodomy that was now illegal, but *any* kind of sex act between two men, even behind closed doors.*

Perhaps the most famous medical text on sexuality in the late Victorian era was the German forensic psychiatrist and university professor Richard von Krafft-Ebing's magnum opus *Psychopathia Sexualis*. If you've heard of Krafft-Ebing, you may be aware that he introduced the terms 'sadism' and 'masochism' to describe the sexual desire for domination and submission respectively, yet another example of how 'normal' sex and pathology are defined by cultural expectations. Masochists were almost always men, Krafft-Ebing said, because the 'passive role' of women in society meant that they 'naturally' connected 'ideas of subjection' to sex and subordination was 'to a

---

* These laws did not tend to prohibit sex acts between women, which were deemed less of a problem – probably because most medical writers thought women had little or no interest in sex.

certain extent a normal manifestation'. It was only in men that such behaviour was abnormal, since it indicated a 'pathological growth of specific feminine mental elements'. Krafft-Ebing even saw domestic violence as potentially normal. 'Among the lower classes of Slavs', he claimed, 'it is said that the wives feel hurt if they are not beaten by their husbands.'[36]

The notion that violence and submission are 'natural' gendered traits has had a long hangover. Not only did a division into male and female sexual habits reinforce a binary model of gender, it also had significant social and legal consequences. Until at least the 1970s, domestic violence was trivialised by police and the courts in many countries, and it wasn't until 1991 that non-consensual sex within marriage became legally regarded as rape in the UK. Gender-based violence was, for far too long, accepted as socially normal, thanks largely to the attitudes of the era in which sexual pathologies were first categorised in medicine.

The main topic of *Psychopathia Sexualis* was not, however, sadism and masochism but homosexuality. By the second edition of 1887, homosexuality had become the definitive perversion for Krafft-Ebing, an emphasis that grew as lay readers began to see themselves in his work and write 'hosts of letters' to the author.[37] As these letters were added to its pages, *Psychopathia Sexualis* grew from a small book of 110 pages and 47 case studies to more than 600 pages with 238 cases in the twelfth German edition of 1903.[38] Some readers found a new way of understanding themselves in Krafft-Ebing's descriptions; others critiqued or opposed the psychiatrist's views. While one middle-class man professed himself tortured by shame and guilt over his 'abnormal condition', 'Dr X.' rejected the idea of cure proposed by Krafft-Ebing.[39] 'The majority of "aunts", like myself', wrote X., 'in no way regret their abnormality, but would be sorry if the condition were to be changed.'[40]

While Krafft-Ebing developed increasing sympathy for the unhappy Urnings who wrote to him, his psychiatric model nonetheless made homosexuality into a pathology. As *Psychopathia Sexualis* grew, the lives and personalities of those engaging in same-sex behaviour came under increasing scrutiny. And, following Krafft-Ebing and his contemporaries, psychiatry remained at the centre of defining 'normal' sexuality for the first half of the twentieth century. These definitions continued to link sexuality with gendered traits. In 1936, psychologists Catharine Cox Miles and Lewis Terman even developed a masculinity–femininity test, which aimed to 'make possible a quantitative estimation of the amount and direction of a subject's deviation from the mean of his or her sex'.[41] While their study began to question the widespread assumption that there was always a link between gendered traits and sexuality, they nonetheless concluded that 'male homosexuals of the passive type as a rule earn markedly feminine scores'.[42]

These stereotypes affected the lives of ordinary people. In the US, efforts to reduce the number of psychiatric casualties by advance screening of recruits in the Second World War proceeded on the basis that homosexuality was a result of neurosis. Recruits could be rejected if they seemed uncomfortable with stripping naked, if they worked as hairdressers or made gestures judged effeminate.[43] Standard questions asked by admission doctors even included the blunt 'Do you like girls?' while official surveys associated normal development in young men with the 'establishment of satisfactory heterosexual relationships'.[44] Between four and five thousand men were rejected by the US Army on the grounds of homosexuality and, during the Second World War, a further 10,000 soldiers were found guilty of occasional homosexual offences.[45]

After the war, a US desire to return to so-called normal was marked by a deeply conservative culture and a renewed focus on family values and pre-war gender roles. Twenty-one states brought in 'sex psychopath' laws, focused on policing behaviour that did not fit these normative standards.[46] People could be convicted for '"nonviolent offenses" such as consensual sodomy, public indecency, patronizing gay bars, touching in public, or cross-dressing'.[47] While laws did eventually change, the idea that homosexuality was a mental illness lingered well beyond the Victorian era. It was not until 1973 that the American Psychiatric Association bowed to pressure from gay rights groups and agreed to remove homosexuality as an illness category from the DSM, and as late as 1990 that the World Health Organization dropped it from the International Classification of Diseases.[48] The associated notion that sexuality was linked to gendered traits also continued to have currency: gay men were assumed to be feminine, lesbians to be 'butch'. This supported an either/or model of sexuality and gender: certain traits were male or female, just as certain people were gay or straight. But things couldn't really be that simple, could they? If other normal traits existed on a scale, then why not sex?

THE DISTRIBUTION OF SEX

One Saturday in December 1891, a quiet marriage ceremony took place in Paddington Registry Office. Henry Havelock Ellis, a thirty-two-year-old physician, married thirty-year-old writer and women's rights activist Edith Lees. The only guests were Ellis's sister Louie and Lees's friends Evelyn and Sybil Brooke. There was no wedding breakfast. While Edith was popular, her new husband hated large gatherings and public speaking. Edith 'mercifully' allowed Havelock to arrive late at the party she threw that afternoon for her numerous friends, so that his 'discomfort was of brief duration'.[49] The next day, the Ellises travelled to Paris. 'Marriage brought no ecstasy,' Havelock Ellis wrote later of his wife, 'but it brought a certain liberation.'[50] Enough that, a year or so later, Edith wrote to Havelock to tell him of her feelings for her friend Claire. The revelation was painful, Havelock later declared, for at the time he had little understanding of 'inborn sexual inversion of character'.[51] Nonetheless he wrote to Edith that 'I am perfectly happy that you should be so close to Claire'.[52] The Ellises agreed to embark upon an open marriage, and homosexuality became one of Havelock's first studies.

Havelock Ellis became 'an authority on sex', a position that amused his intimate female friends greatly, he recalled, given 'how small my experience was'.[53] Between 1897 and 1908, this quiet and reclusive doctor, philosopher, artist, poet, musician, scientist and eugenicist published six volumes of *Studies in the Psychology of Sex*. Ellis's interest in sex 'in fairly healthy and normal people' took a huge step away from the previous emphasis on pathology and law.[54] His work rejected the psychiatric view of homosexuality; it also questioned the idea of same-sex attraction as gender inversion. 'Masculine traits were indeed not obvious in Edith,' Ellis recalled, concluding somewhat patronisingly that 'she was not really man at all in any degree, but always woman, boy, and child'.[55]

Female homosexuals received far greater prominence in Ellis's writings than elsewhere, largely thanks to the input of Edith and her friends. Edith Ellis became one of the case studies in *Sexual Inversion*: Miss H., a thirty-year-old who had first experienced sexual interest in other girls at the age of four.[56] As an adult, Miss H. found 'sexual satisfaction in tenderly touching, caressing and kissing the loved one's body'. 'Homosexual love', Miss H. declared, 'is morally right when it is really part of a person's nature.' It was not, however, acceptable 'as a mere makeshift, or expression of sensuality, in normal women'.[57]

This theme – of the moral importance of love, and the inborn, essential nature of homosexuality – appeared throughout Ellis's work and case studies. Unlike Krafft-Ebing's diseased inverts, *Sexual Inversion* presented the homosexual as the ideal, civilised person, with strong morals and an immense power of self-control. It was society that made same-sex encounters seem abnormal, inhibiting the efforts of Edith Ellis or John Addington Symonds (Ellis's collaborator on *Sexual Inversion*) to form 'permanent ties' with their lovers.

When Havelock Ellis was writing in the early twentieth century, ideas of normal sexuality were also influenced by Freud. Freud had initially focused his attention on perversion and pathology, with sexual experiences in child-hood (including abuse) used to explain adult neuroses. In 1899, however, he proposed the existence of a normal childhood sexual drive, or libido, and in his 1905 essays on the theory of sexuality he began to view what he had called 'aberrations' (like homosexuality) as variations within nature.[58] Yet Freud's model, as we have already seen, was developmental. Like masturbation, homosexuality was a stage in sexual development, with heterosexual vaginal sex as the 'normal' act towards which every other form of sexual activity progressed. Even though homosexual desires were normal in children, in adults Freud thought they showed arrested development, making homosexuality a form of neurosis. Ellis had a slightly different, but no less normative take: loving, monogamous bonds between two individuals formed the normal where sex was concerned, and anything that departed from this ideal was a perversion. Both Freud and Ellis also saw sexuality as absolute and unchanging. It wasn't until after the Second World War that Alfred Kinsey shifted the notion of normal sex yet again.

There's a memorable scene in the 2004 film *Kinsey* in which Alfred Kinsey (Liam Neeson) and his colleague Clyde Martin (Peter Sarsgaard) are relaxing in their hotel room, midway through a trip to collect sex interviews. They're discussing the Kinsey scale, the idea that sexuality is a relative and fluid concept. Most people, according to Kinsey, fall somewhere between 0 (entirely heterosexual) and 6 (entirely homosexual). 'I guess I'm about a three, huh?' Martin states, before asking his colleague, 'How about you?' 'I suppose I've been a one or two most of my life,' Kinsey replies thoughtfully. 'And now?' Martin presses. 'Probably three,' Kinsey replies, before the pair start to kiss. In real life, Kinsey filmed himself, colleagues and friends having sex in the attic of his home, a personal devotion to his work that for some lends a touch of suspicion to his conclusions. Regardless of his motivation, Kinsey's scale was the first attempt to move beyond a binary model of human sexuality – encompassing such a wide range of variation that no level of homosexual or heterosexual experience could be regarded as definitively normal or abnormal.

Between 1938 and 1963, the former entomologist and his colleagues at the Institute for Sex Research gathered a staggering 18,216 detailed sex histories of American people.[59] Like Ellis, Kinsey wanted to look at 'normal' sex, but his method of doing so was quantitative not qualitative. By taking thousands of detailed histories, Kinsey aimed to uncover what types of behaviour really were statistically common in American society, and not what was dictated by social codes. He thus tried to move away from the value structures used in other surveys, where questions were framed to indicate disapproval of, say, masturbation or homosexuality.[60] Rather than asking if someone had ever masturbated, interviewers asked how old the interviewee was when masturbation began.[61]

It was commonly believed, Kinsey and his colleagues noted, that homosexual and heterosexual men were different physically, mentally and emotionally. Gay men were assumed to have fine skins, delicate movements, high-pitched voices, to be artistically sensitive, emotionally unbalanced, and interested in the arts. However, the 'world is not to be divided into sheep and goats,' Kinsey wrote.

'Only the human mind invents categories and tries to force facts into separated pigeon-holes.'[62] Kinsey's data disproved nearly a century of assumption that there was a clear difference between two discrete populations: heterosexuals and homosexuals. Indeed, 'a considerable portion of the population, perhaps the major portion of the male population, has at least some homosexual experience'.[63] Far from being abnormal, the Kinsey study proved that same-sex acts were a common and 'significant part of human sexual activity'.[64]

The overturning of the gender inversion model of homosexuality was important. This model assumed that any population could be divided into simple binary categories: male and female; heterosexual and homosexual; normal and abnormal. Even for Havelock Ellis, bisexuality was suspicious because it implied the 'makeshift' of which Edith Ellis so disapproved: by not fitting a binary model of sex or gender, bisexuality implied that someone was denying the feelings of their true 'soul' or seeking out carnal pleasure over love. Once again, this set of norms has had a long legacy. Think of the character of Ferdy in the 1990s TV series *This Life*, constantly accused of being scared to come out of the closet because no one could believe he might be attracted to his wife *and* to other men.

Kinsey rejected a binary model of sex and viewed sexuality on a scale unrelated to gender. As a biologist he saw variation as a positive thing. There is no such thing as abnormal sexual behaviour, he told his students at Indiana University, for 'nearly all of the so-called sexual perversions fall within the range of biologic normality'.[65] Even Kinsey, though, couldn't escape normative judgements entirely. His determination to reveal the truth about 'normal' American sex meant that his published studies emphasised groups thought to *be* the most normal: white, middle-class college graduates. While this was partly intentional, in that Kinsey aimed to stop critics assuming that all 'deviance' could be attributed to minority groups – in actual fact, patterns of sexual experience for Black and white men were similar within each social class – it nonetheless served to perpetuate the idea that white America was the normal standard.[66]

People continued to compare themselves to preconceived norms, of course. 'On the whole,' respondents to a British survey of 1949 were asked to consider, 'would you say that you yourself are sexually normal, or not?' Aiming to record the sexual attitudes and habits of the British public, this survey by Mass Observation was nicknamed 'Little Kinsey' by researchers and readers alike.*

Answers varied enormously. Some respondents thought that they were normal whatever social conventions were: 'For an homosexual, I am normal,' declared a twenty-five-year-old man. Mass Observation's coders disagreed with his judgement, pencilling a red '2' for homosexual on to his returned survey instead of the usual '0' for normal. Normal, as so often, was more about prevailing social assumptions than about individual identity. Two men who declared themselves over-sexed were both categorised as abnormal, even though one thought he was 'normal on the whole' while the other said he definitely wasn't. A twenty-six-year-old lab assistant said he wasn't normal because he

---

* Formed in 1937 by left-wing researchers, Mass Observation intended to create 'an anthropology of ourselves': a study of everyday life in Britain based on surveys, diaries and personal documents gathered by a mix of voluntary respondents and paid researchers. The members of their panel were largely (but not exclusively) middle class, and men considerably outnumbered women.

regretted not having a promiscuous youth; his survey wasn't coded at all.[67] Despite the efforts of 1940s social scientists to decide if British people were sexually normal, their codes couldn't capture the huge breadth of variation in attitudes and experiences. And individuals, too, questioned the idea of a normal standard for sex. One forty-eight-year-old man professed himself normal 'but at the same time must admit that I have no knowledge of what the norm might be'. 'Can you define normal?' asked another participant.

One in five respondents to Little Kinsey reported some form of homosexual experience.[68] British men and women, however, were more similar than their American counterparts: 21 per cent of men and 19 per cent of women reported some form of sexual relations with the same sex.[69] Admittedly, the female sample was based on very small numbers: less than 100 surveys were completed by women compared to over 300 by men. Yet it nonetheless showed that homosexual sex, while not a majority experience, was not unusual. It was also not necessarily something that people thought abnormal, even though it remained illegal in Britain at the time. Two-thirds of men and three-quarters of women who had had a homosexual experience deemed themselves sexually normal. And while a quarter of women who had had same-sex encounters thought themselves abnormal, so too did a quarter of women who had never had a homosexual experience.

Others grudgingly admitted a point of departure between their own lives and social expectation. 'I suppose [I'm] not normal,' a forty-year-old civil servant bemoaned. 'The convention is of sexual intercourse only with the opposite sex.' However, he wished that his own experiences 'were more universal'. If, he thought, society took 'a more understanding view of such members of the community who are like myself', then 'more stable and permanent relationships could be fostered'. A woman who described herself as both homosexual and abnormal, meanwhile, had no sexual experiences at all to recount. 'I know I am not sexually normal,' she explained, 'since I have lived to be 30 without ever falling in love or being made love to, nor having any of the normal desires for love-making, marriage or children.' Her shyness prevented her from trying to initiate a sexual relationship with either a man or a woman, though having read Radclyffe Hall's lesbian novel *The Well of Loneliness*, she thought she probably could make love to a woman. 'So it looks as if I shall die celibate,' she concluded surprisingly brusquely, 'though I don't let it worry me nor brood about it.'[70]

By the time the British National Survey of Sexual Attitudes and Lifestyles was published in 1994, the next major British sex survey after Little Kinsey, homosexuality was no longer either illegal or medically pathologised (officially, at least). But strangely, *fewer* people seemed to be having homosexual experiences. Just 5.3 per cent of men and 2.8 per cent of women reported ever having had sex with someone of the same gender. By 1999–2001, when the age of consent had finally been equalised for homosexual and heterosexual sex, this rose to 8.4 per cent of men and 9.7 per cent of women, less than half the rate recorded by Little Kinsey in 1949.[71] Beyond the stigma of the AIDS epidemic and the high refusal rate of the survey, there may be other reasons for the seemingly stark decline in same-sex experiences.[72] Even though it was no longer classed as a crime or a psychiatric illness, gay sex could still be presented as morally dubious: think of George Michael's arrest in a public toilet in 1998 when so-called 'lewd' encounters in public bathrooms and parks became a media moral panic.[73] The gay rights movement, while achieving many things, also contributed to an essentialisation of homosexuality. When I was a teenager, no one talked about a moving scale of sexual desire and behaviour, as Alfred Kinsey had done, they were too busy looking for the 'gay gene'. To be gay or straight was simply what you *were*, the way you were born.

Having grown up in this era of essentialisation, the surveys of the 1940s and 1950s – Kinsey and Little Kinsey alike – seem oddly liberating, despite the legal repression, moral attitudes and individual guilt that surrounded them. I suppose part of me had assumed that people in the past felt invariably trapped, made miserable by furtive same-sex encounters and the absence of meaningful relationships. Yet, from Fanny and Stella to Little Kinsey, many people have engaged in active and enjoyable sex lives – and held long-term relationships – with members of the same sex. In Dr X.'s small town of 30,000 inhabitants, he told Krafft-Ebing in the 1890s, he personally knew around 120 'aunts', and overall had met 'thousands of such individuals'.[74] During the First World War, Vera 'Jack' Holme had love affairs with numerous women. Nurses Lady Hermione Blackwood and Cathlin du Sautoy, who lived and worked together in the same war, adopted two French orphans, jointly bringing them up in Hampstead. Of course, not everyone enjoyed the same advantages; a privileged background often served as protection. Yet it is striking that, in the Little Kinsey survey, the number of unhappy 'sexually abnormal' married women far outnumbered those people who worried about their experiences with same-sex partners. Women, it seems, have been judged by particularly punishing standards where sexual normalcy is concerned.

LIKE A VIRGIN

The ironic, knowing, yet oddly innocent 'Like a Virgin' proved a smash hit for pop icon Madonna in 1984: her first American number-one single. It was released two years after my little sister was born, when I was five, so it wasn't until the early 1990s that the two of us became obsessed with Madonna's music – and her life, which seemed a world away from the suburban bunkbeds we plastered with her picture. After the release of *Erotica* in 1992 my sister spent all her holiday money on a biography of our idol. It made for interesting reading. 'Mummy says Madonna's not a nice person because she slept with all those men,' my eleven-year-old sister wrote frankly to our granny, 'but *I* think she's just generous.' Our interpretation of how much sex is too much depends on all sorts of things. How many different partners has someone had? What do we think about that person otherwise? How do their actions compare with our own lives and experiences? And, perhaps most tellingly, what is that person's gender?

My generation was brought up with the idea that, sexually speaking, 'men are from Mars, women are from Venus'.[75] Men demand physical sex; women want an emotional connection, or so goes the stereotype. Historically, this stark distinction between men and women is relatively recent. In the sixteenth and seventeenth centuries, women were presented in literature and medicine as lustful, bawdy, passionate and sexually active, even though, contradictorily, chastity was a much prized and policed trait in young ladies.[76] Female sexual pleasure could be positive, connected to a woman's fertility. Even a woman's sex organs were not considered fundamentally different from a man's. This 'one sex' model of humankind, as historian Thomas Laqueur calls it, held that the female genitalia were an inverted or undescended version of the male's – different in appearance, not in kind.[77]

In the nineteenth century, however, women's bodies and minds became seen as fundamentally different from those of men. After the French Revolution of 1789, the ideal woman was increasingly presented as passionless, passive and pure, unsuited to physical or mental employment – her sole purpose pregnancy and motherhood.[78] It was in this context that the so-called 'double standard' emerged, a sexual divide that has haunted women ever since. 'The majority of women (happily for them)', as Victorian doctor William Acton put it in 1865, 'are not very much troubled with sexual feeling of any kind.' While Acton's words were intended to reassure impotent men, and other doctors were not quite so sure that women had no interest in sex at all, most agreed that women's sexual desire was limited.[79] 'What men are habitually,' Acton concluded, making a distinction that has threaded through popular opinion even into the present day, 'women are only exceptionally.'[80] Men think about sex every seven seconds, as the urban myth goes (except it turns out they don't).[81]

Women who did not fit with this passionless 'standard' were nymphomaniacs; they had an abnormal desire for sex. This expansive condition had many symptoms, including lewd behaviour, masturbation and promiscuity, as well as 'adultery, flirting, being divorced, or feeling more passionate than their husbands'.[82] In 1850s Boston, when Mrs B.'s husband was unable to keep up with her desire for nightly sex, her gynaecologist recommended temporary separation and a host of privations to limit sensuality. 'If she continued in her present habits of indulgence,' he warned, 'it would probably become necessary to send her to an asylum.'[83] Excessive sex was thought to be a problem for everyone, but the male form of this condition – satyriasis – was deemed milder and less common.[84]

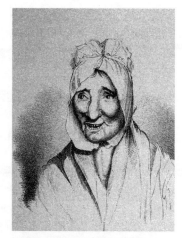

Print from Alexander Morison's *Physiognomy of Mental Diseases* (1843), showing 'an elderly female, in whom lascivious ideas predominated, constituting the variety termed Nymphomania'.

Of course, it was not only husbands who worried about their wives' failure to follow social convention; women themselves worried too. Some sought out the help of physicians or were forced to submit to cures for their sexual desire by friends and family members. In America, surgical removal of the clitoris (clitoridectomy) was an accepted treatment for masturbation well into the twentieth century.[85] The same practice acquired a dubious reputation in

Britain after the discrediting of its main advocate, gynae-cologist Isaac Baker Brown, in 1867. Baker Brown was accused of self-advertising – which smacked of quackery to Victorian medical practitioners – and failing to obtain the consent of his patients before mutilating them.[86] Despite Baker Brown's expulsion from the Obstetrical Society and death in 1873, clitoridectomy in Britain did not entirely die with him.[87]

Women who were not subjected to surgical treatment also struggled with the weight of society's demands. Nancy Jessie Joy was twenty-one years old and working as head stillroom maid at a house in Pall Mall when she was admitted to Bethlem Royal Hospital in 1888. Discharged just five days earlier, Joy attempted suicide after 'seduc-tion': a popular Victorian euphemism for pre-marital sex in women. She had still been depressed when she left the hospital and had the idea that 'if she became "ruined" a change would come over her mind'. Nancy was 'accosted by a gentleman' and 'allowed him to have intercourse with her', the doctors wrote, but 'now feels she is going to hell and wants to hurry this on'.

This 'ruination' weighed heavily on Nancy Joy's mind. Discharged again six months later, she wrote to the hospi-tal in 1891. Now engaged to be married, Joy did not want to tell her fiancé about her past. Distressed and confused, the young woman sought help and advice from her former doctors, telling them of her remorse and 'the bitter tears I shed at times when alone'. Even though 'in my sane mind not an impure thought enters my mind', Nancy Joy had spent years worrying over her state, and now simply wanted a final answer. 'Am I really ruined or not?' she queried.

'If I am I will never marry, no man shall reproach.' Poor 'ruined' Nancy didn't marry her fiancé; when she returned to Bethlem a few years later, she was still single.[88]

Other women campaigned on behalf of those like Nancy Joy, most famously Josephine Butler, who spearheaded protests against the Contagious Diseases Acts.* Rather than struggle to convince men to treat women differently, Butler decided to seek out and support these women herself. This crusade was personal. Following the unexpected death of her young daughter Eva in 1866, Butler threw herself into this work with a missionary zeal, 'possessed with an irresistible desire to go forth and find some pain keener than my own'.[89] Women – Marion, Katie, Margaret, Emma and Laura – were invited from the streets to live out their final days in Butler's home.[90] Their common story was that they had 'been trampled under the feet of men, as the mire in the streets'.[91] Butler's tales of these women's woes were marked by two things: a desire to reclaim them as innocent passive victims and an avenging fury at the men who had 'trampled' them.

While Butler and her colleagues did not refute the idea that biological differences between men and women made men more interested in sex, it was not long before others began to openly protest this assumption. Marie Stopes's *Married Love* (1918) was a bestseller, improving the sex lives of countless couples by emphasising the importance of

* First passed in 1864, the Acts aimed to reduce the rate of venereal disease in the armed forces by allowing the arrest and forced medical examination of any woman suspected of being a prostitute. Butler and her colleagues called the exam an 'instrumental rape' and railed against the double standard that it implied. For the full story, see Judith R. Walkowitz, *Prostitution and Victorian Society: Women, Class, and the State* (Cambridge: Cambridge University Press, 1980).

female, as well as male, desire. When a workhouse lawyer wrote to Stopes to insist that the 'normal man's sexual passion is stronger than the normal woman's', Stopes disagreed. 'I do not believe that the normal man's sex needs are stronger than the normal woman's,' she replied. 'The *average* man's undoubtedly are, owing to the utterly false repression of the woman's.'[92] Despite her enthusiasm for the biological racism of eugenics, Stopes insisted that differences between men's and women's sexual desires were socially determined, *not* biological.

Kinsey came to similar conclusions. Men and women were not fundamentally different sexually, the former entomologist insisted, though he thought they did differ psychologically. Women showed greater sexual variation than men, but it was variation itself that remained the 'most persistent reality in human behavior'.[93] This meant that there were greater differences between individual humans than there were between men and women as groups: yet more evidence supporting the uncoupling of sexuality from gender. Kinsey's view of gender as a spectrum had definite limits, however. In the late 1940s, trans activist Louise Lawrence tried to convince Kinsey that trans people were 'much more common than most of us, even prominent doctors are willing or able to admit'.[94] Yet, as historian Katie Sutton explains, Kinsey's emphasis on the physical basis of sex in orgasm meant that, although broadly sympathetic, he did not support surgery for trans people.[95]

The Little Kinsey study suggested that, in Britain in 1949, many young, middle-class people were sexually active before marriage, but double standards still prevailed. Women who had children out of wedlock were frowned upon, sometimes even institutionalised, and the men who fathered those children all but forgotten. Women who were sexually assaulted might be shunned, assumed to be to blame for attracting attention in the first place.[96] Some men taking the survey made their reliance on this double standard clear. 'If I'm going around just for a good time I don't mind taking a girl,' a twenty-three-year-old builder's labourer told the Little Kinsey interviewer, 'but if I was going with a girl I was wanting to marry I wouldn't touch her.'[97] A twenty-year-old Londoner similarly stressed that, even though he himself had had sex with ten different girls, he would no longer want to marry his fiancée if she agreed to his advances.[98] 'I was determined that I could never marry a girl that would allow intercourse between us before marriage,' a twenty-nine-year-old motor engineer agreed. 'I had great difficulty in finding one, but I did, and I married her.'[99]

This hypocrisy continued through the 1960s, the contradictory decade that began with the obscenity trial of the novel *Lady Chatterley's Lover* in the UK and the launch of the contraceptive pill. While 'the pill' has been seen as a liberating force for female sexual desire, at first it was only available to married

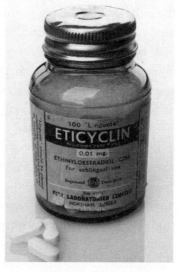

Bottle of 'Eticyclin' (1954–71), an early combined oestrogen and progestin contraceptive pill.

women. The first birth control clinics for unmarried women in the UK were launched in 1964 and were 'constantly accused of encouraging promiscuity'.[100] While sexual pleasure in women was no longer automatically a sign of mental illness, levels of female sexual activity remained carefully monitored, in psychiatry as well as reproductive medicine.

In the US, eighteen-year-old Susanna Kaysen was described as 'promiscuous' when she was admitted to McLean Psychiatric Hospital in 1967. She had to be sent to hospital, the admitting psychiatrist warned, because otherwise she 'might kill [her]self or get pregnant'.[101] Judging by the hospital population around her, Kaysen later noted, compulsive promiscuity was a common diagnosis for young American women in the 1960s. 'How many girls do you think a seventeen-year-old boy would have to screw to earn the label "compulsively promiscuous"?' she asked. 'Probably in the fifteen-to-twenty range, would be my guess – if they ever put that label on boys, which I don't recall their doing.' She finishes with an unanswered question. 'And for seventeen-year-old girls, how many boys?'[102] The definition of too much sex relied heavily on gendered norms.

'Promiscuous' remained a dangerous label for women in the later twentieth century. In 1980, for example, newspapers and magazines around the world reported on a Swedish study that linked promiscuity in women with higher rates of cervical cancer. Except it didn't really. The study suggested that a cancer-causing bacterial agent (later identified as the human papillomavirus or HPV) had been found in semen. Mysteriously, rather than conclude that this might require treating the men who were spreading the bacteria, or advising people to use condoms, the conclusion of most newspaper articles was that female promiscuity was the problem.[103] In addition to these gendered stereotypes, Black women had to contend with an added layer of racist assumptions. A colleague once told me that she was terrified of getting cervical cancer as a teenager in the 1980s, because she was told Black girls were at greater risk. It was only years later that she discovered that this 'risk' was based on the medical establishment's assumption that Black women were more promiscuous than white women, a racist stereotype that can be traced back to at least the seventeenth century.[104]

When I became a teenager in the 1990s, normal sex was a difficult balance for young women. To be nervous about sex was to be frigid; to know too much about it was to be a slut or a slag. To be on the pill too young was dubious, yet to accidentally get pregnant was a moral failing. 'This country would be a better place if women just kept their legs together!' my classmate announced – echoing her Tory dad – when I mentioned that my sixteen-year-old cousin had had a baby. Why it was the sole responsibility of women to improve the country went unquestioned. Single mothers had replaced unwed mothers as the pariahs of the Thatcherite state, compounding the difficulties in their lives. Concerns about teen sexuality threaded through girls' magazines of the 1990s and 2000s too. While these magazines ran features that supported 'young women's agentic quest for sexual experience' and presented sexual experimentation as 'normal', agony aunts silenced female readers' desires by emphasising their lack of readiness for sex.[105] A different kind of waiting was suggested for those whose desires did not fit heterosexual expectation:

'Be careful not to label yourself as anything just yet' was a warning meted out only to those who expressed a preference for the same sex.[106]

In 2016, extra-marital dating site IllicitEncounters.com carried out a survey of its members' expectations in a new partner. They found that both men and women thought the ideal number of prior partners in their new lover was a nicely rounded ten, although straight men remained marginally more wary of women with a higher number of previous lovers. 'If we had conducted this poll ten years ago,' a spokesman for the site claimed, 'men would have expected a potential partner to have slept with far fewer people.'[107] Was this statement true? Had the double standard really lingered so long, even among people presumably more accepting of sex outside relationships? It seems possible. In many countries – though not all – enjoying sex is now expected of everyone, within and outside marriage, regardless of sexuality or gender identity. Scratch beneath the surface, though, and gendered expectations remain. It's women, not men, who are censured for the size of their families or for being single parents. And the way women dress or behave on a night out is still raised in the media and courtrooms across the Western world as a defence against accusations of sexual assault. Victims of rape – who are disproportionately female – are 'uniquely vulnerable' to being blamed for their assault, explained three psychologists in 2019, something that doesn't happen with other interpersonal crimes.[108] The link between 'normal' sex and gender, and the double standard it has supported, is something that we're still struggling to shrug off.

WHAT IS (NORMAL) SEX ANYWAY?

A few years ago we had a big restructure at work. As a junior manager, I was encouraged to read a short text about supporting a team through change. For some reason, this was explained through the medium of penguins. These penguins all had different skills and abilities and had to work as a group in a complicated move from their melting ice cap to safety. While the characters were all penguins, they were humanised in a range of ways. They had jobs, and tools and language. They were also, without exception, in monogamous heterosexual relationships or nuclear families, and frequently had gender stereotyped traits (even if the authors made sure that some girl penguins were leaders and engineers). It wasn't really relevant to the message, but it irritated me nonetheless. I moaned about it to a friend, and she pulled a face. 'Oh no,' she empathised, 'they're not *heteronormative* penguins, are they?'

The term 'heteronormative' was coined in 1991 by Michael Warner[109] and has since been used to describe a range of ways in which society is policed along the lines of gender and sexuality.[110] It emphasises the way heterosexuality has been and is privileged as a category, and how this is often accompanied by gendered forms of bias or exclusion. There was no need for the authors of a management guide to put all their penguins into heterosexual nuclear families. This detail was hardly relevant to the ice cap disaster project, and it's not even true that all *penguins* behave in heterosexual and monogamous ways.

This may sound like a trivial example, but those heteronormative penguins are just one of countless instances across history and culture – some everyday, some more sinister – in which a certain form of sex is repeatedly emphasised as normal simply by the exclusion of any variation. We see it in books, in films, in the newspapers or on TV. To be heterosexual is undefined, oddly invisible despite being everywhere. Only fictional characters who do not fit this presumed norm are identified by their sexuality or gender identity. And so it has been for a century and a half: a certain type of sex – in association with a binary model of gender – is presumed to be normal, and everything else is defined in relation to it. Difference is erased, leading to the mistaken impression among those who do fit this picture that everyone is the same, and marginalising all those who cannot see themselves in the lives of a huddle of heteronormative penguins. Yet, as the Kinsey study showed, even in the 1940s it was not all that usual to be exclusively heterosexual.

The way judgements about normal sex have shifted over the centuries reminds us just how central cultural attitudes are to defining sexual norms, and how many people have been imprisoned, excluded, blackmailed and worse for not fitting into them. Many of us today would consider masturbation both usual and natural; yet for centuries, self-love was the *most* abnormal of sexual acts. The stigma of the solitary vice remained long after the damaging physical effects of the practice were proven to be a myth. Homosexuality, meanwhile, was medically classified as an abnormal way of being only in the late nineteenth century. Heterosexual sex became the norm *because* of the rising interest in this so-called pathology. The very term 'heterosexual' was introduced in gay literature, while medical texts in the nineteenth and twentieth centuries began to use vaginal intercourse as a yardstick for measuring the relative normality of other kinds of sex act.

This comparative view of sex remains in place, to some extent. If I asked you how many sexual partners you'd had, how would you go about counting? Would you encompass 'any form of lovemaking' as the Little Kinsey survey put it in 1949? Or would you count only the times that came closest to a penetrative norm? Some respondents to Little Kinsey found themselves frustrated by such rigid definitions of sex. A fifty-five-year-old woman strongly objected to the question 'Have you ever gone in for love-making which stopped short only of intercourse?' 'I find this question needs amplifying,' she added in a note. 'I have often had love-passages which did not go on to intercourse, but there was no policy of stopping short.'[111] With six prior partners (five men and one woman), she didn't lack for experience. Lovemaking, she insisted, was not simply a preliminary to intercourse. Sex was not a matter of biology but differed for different people; it required negotiation and compromise, communication and learned skill.

The question isn't just what's normal, then, but what is sex at all?

5

IS THIS A NORMAL
WAY TO FEEL?

It was a blazing hot summer day in 1986. Or maybe it wasn't that hot. All my childhood summers seem to blur into one long hazy memory of blistering sunshine, day after day – with the occasional sudden downpour whenever we tried to have a family barbecue. There were hosepipe bans, and the grass around the edge of the tarmacked school playground died. I remember being fascinated by the way the dry, bare earth cracked into a pattern of hexagons and wondered if this was what a desert looked like. There must, of course, have been plenty of days that didn't fit this pattern but, unremarkable as they were to a seven-year-old, they've long since faded from my mind.

That day, somewhere towards the end of the school holidays, didn't seem remarkable either at first. Mum said she had to go out and sent me and my little sister to play with the boys next door. It wasn't unusual for us to spend half the day next door. Dad even put a gate between the two back gardens so we could all come and go more easily for games of football, or spies, or the Famous Five: whatever it was we were into that summer. My sister and I didn't even think anything of it when Matthew turned gravely to me. 'I think one of your friends has just died,' he said, with all the gravity a six-year-old could muster. 'But that doesn't matter, you'll still have me and all your other friends.'

I was older and wiser than Matthew. I thought he was making this up or had misunderstood something he had heard. So I don't remember being overly concerned when Mum came home soon after and called us inside, into a house that seemed cool and dark after the sunny garden.

It turned out that Matthew was right. He'd overheard my mum telling his mum that my best friend, Katie, had been hit by a lorry while out on her bike and died instantly. Mum couldn't quite believe it when she got the phone call and, in shock, she'd gone round to Katie's house to make sure.

When Mum told us the news, to our surprise my sister and I both burst out laughing. It was a confusing response to something even four-year-old Alison was old enough to know was sad. Confusing but totally normal, Mum told us, as we cried later over plastic mugs of squash and bourbon biscuits. Mum told us she had laughed as a child when the family dog died and felt terrible about it. It's the shock, she said. When you hear unexpected bad news, it's an automatic reaction. It doesn't mean you don't care, that you aren't upset.

Emotions can be especially confusing for young children. What do our feelings mean, and how do we express or explain them to others? In infant school, Miss Taylor once read the class of five-year-olds a story about a little girl who stole chocolates from her sister. I cried and cried, but when the teacher asked me what was wrong I couldn't find the words to explain. In the end I just told Miss Taylor I was hungry. I knew that wasn't the right way to describe what I was feeling, but the sensation was a little bit like hunger so that explanation had to do.

But it's not only children who find it hard to define emotion. Psychologists and psychiatrists – and, before them, philosophers and theologists – have long struggled to pinpoint what exactly our emotions are. In 1884, American psychologist William James famously suggested that emotions are biological reactions to an event. For James, we don't cry because we are sad but are sad because we cry. Our reaction is immediate, impulsive and unconscious, and it is only later that we label it as a feeling.[1] Since James's time, the way we understand and talk about emotion has changed further. Psychoanalysts held that our feelings needed to be interpreted; behaviourists that they were evidence of unconscious conditioning.

More recently, neurobiologists have tried to locate specific emotions in different parts of the brain. The best-known example is the pinpointing of 'fear' in the amygdala, a tiny almond-shaped collection of cells near the base of the brain. The amygdala triggers the well-known 'fight-or-flight' response to a threat. Yet there remain a whole host of culturally and individually determined questions, even in this neurological model. What do we perceive as threatening in the first place? How do we experience fear? How do we explain it to ourselves and to others? And what is our actual eventual response? All these things change depending on history, culture and individual circumstance: you might be terrified of spiders, but I might think they look adorably vulnerable with their long, spindly legs (I do, I've been official spider remover in every friendship group since Brownie camp).

Despite these questions, most researchers into the mind have assumed that emotions exist, a universal aspect of human life. But would it surprise you to know that until recently the Tibetan language didn't even have a word for 'emotion'? Eventually, Tibetan teachers were asked for the translation so often that a word was coined, though it has only slowly gathered meaning for many Tibetans. This is not to say that people in Tibet do not feel, nor that they don't have names for specific types of feeling. They simply had not grouped them into one concept: emotions.[2]

This is also the case historically. Before 1830, English-language writers on the mind used a wide range of terms for feeling, many of which borrowed from religious language: passions, affections and sentiments. There were significant differences between categories. Passions were impulsive and instinctive; sentiments required experience or education to develop. As Louis Antoine de Saint-Just, one of the architects of the Reign of Terror during the French Revolution, put it, 'We must not confuse the sentiments of the soul with the passions. The first are a gift of nature and the principle of social life. The others are the fruit of usurpation and the principles of savage life.'[3]

By 1850, historian Thomas Dixon has shown, 'emotion' had become the favoured scientific category swallowing up very different feelings, from the simple passion of rage to the complex sentiment of sympathy.[4] Of course, other terms for human feeling continued to be used. However, by grouping a wide range of ideas under the heading of 'the emotions', Victorian writers newly assumed that anger and love, or fear and compassion, functioned in a similar way, both physically and mentally.

Viewing our feelings as emotions also meant that more attention was paid to the balance of these traits. As the nineteenth century progressed, psychologists, psychiatrists and other scientists tried to measure human emotion. They began to wonder what a normal level of feeling was, and how to define it. What did it mean if someone felt too much? Do we need to worry if we feel too little? Are there particular emotions that we should or should not feel? And how ought we to express these feelings? The guidelines for feeling are even more complex than the ways we monitor a normal body or mind since, to this day, no one has agreed what emotions actually are.

BROKEN HEARTS

Grief characterised my childhood after Katie died and for a long time I had recurring nightmares about her death. This emotion has been at the centre of modern concern about normal feelings ever since 2013, when the fifth edition of the DSM – the American manual of psychiatric diagnosis – was reported by the press as stating that more than two weeks of grief after the death of a loved one constituted mental illness.* As anyone who has lost someone close will tell you, grief can be a lengthy and complex process. As a

* This wasn't exactly what the manual said. To be specific, it simply removed bereavement as an excluding factor for diagnosing depression. Any intense melancholy lasting more than a fortnight and interfering with daily life, including grief, can now be diagnosed as depression.

seven-year-old, my life continued. I went to school. I carried on playing football with the boys next door. I made new friends. I certainly didn't feel sad all or even most of the time. But I became quick to cry at any perceived slight and mistrustful of the permanency of other people's feelings for me. 'I don't have a best friend,' I told everyone when I started secondary school. 'Best friends just die or leave you.' Was this 'normal'? Is that even a useful question to ask? We have the right to have our grief accepted, but of course we also have the right to try to ease the pain, by medical, spiritual or other means.

It is not, after all, new for grief to be seen as unhealthy, although in past centuries it was more often regarded as physically dangerous. On 26 March 1667, thirty-four-year-old London civil servant Samuel Pepys wrote in his famous diary that he got up 'with a sad heart in reference to my mother, of whose death I undoubtedly expect to hear the next post, if not of my father's also, who by his pain as well as his grief for her is very ill'.[5] The following day Pepys received news of his mother's death, and he and his wife wept heartily. Despite the intensity of his feelings, Pepys's father did survive for more than another decade. Yet the fear expressed by his son that his father's grief might prove fatal was understandable. In Pepys's time, the weekly London Bills of Mortality published all causes of death across the city. Grief was the most deadly emotion in its pages: between 1629 and 1660, more than 350 people were recorded as having died of grief (considerably more than the mere thirty who died of fright).[6]

Today, we might take this link between feelings and the body as metaphorical. Yet in the seventeenth and

eighteenth centuries, it was believed the heart could literally break, expand or contract as a result of excessive
feeling. Emotional and physical health were intimately
connected.[7] This lingered into the Victorian era, by which
time all emotions could be classed as pathological. Violent
emotion can cause haemorrhage and heart attacks, French
psychologist Charles Féré said in 1892. Fear could 'turn' the
blood, while intense sadness caused obesity, digestive disorders and increased the likelihood of infection.[8] Emotion
caused more ill effects on the body than all other mental
impulses combined, according to British psychiatrist Daniel
Hack Tuke.[9]

There are also more recent links between emotions and
our biology. While in some cases science has disproved the
causation of physical ailments by feelings – as in the isolation of the bacterium causing 'stress'-induced stomach
ulcers in 1984 – in other cases the reverse has been found,
continuing centuries of worry over the connection between
our physical health and abnormal emotional states. Cardi-
ologists have linked heightened emotion to sudden collapses
in heart rhythm, which can even prove fatal.[10] And we
are all constantly warned about the connection between
emotional stress and high blood pressure – although not,
perhaps, how to actually manage this in our hectic lives.

This does not, however, mean that all strong feelings
have always been seen as unhealthy or abnormal. In the
eighteenth century, intense sentiment was a marker of
good character and education. Wealthy, literate Europeans
wanted to be the 'man of feeling' described by Scottish
novelist Henry Mackenzie in 1771, and expressions of profound grief were an intrinsic part of this. No sentimental

story was more praised at the time – or more vilified by later generations – than Johann Wolfgang von Goethe's *The Sorrows of Young Werther*, first published in 1774. The German novella follows the infatuation of young artist Werther with the beautiful, intelligent, loving Lotte in the fictional village of Wahlheim. The extremes of Werther's passion and unrequited love eventually lead to his suicide. Goethe's narrator played the role of editor of Werther's letters, allowing the author to reflect on the emotions of his literary creation. 'You cannot deny your admiration and love for his spirit and character,' he told his reader, suggesting that those who shared Werther's pain could 'draw consolation from his sorrows'.[11] Published at the peak of literary sentimentalism, Goethe's book became a bestseller across Europe. According to later writers, it also sparked an epidemic of suicides.[12]

In the decades after *The Sorrows of Young Werther* was published, a pronounced shift took place in the way both tragic sentiment and suicide were seen. By 1829, such heightened emotion was viewed as increasingly dubious: a sign of instability. The age of sentiment, it was now claimed, had caused the French Revolution. In 1893, the American philosopher and mathematician Charles Sanders Peirce, despite defending sentimentalism, bluntly asserted that 'it brought about the Reign of Terror', during which more than 15,000 people were sentenced to death.[13] Strong emotions were now politically as well as physically dubious. This may seem an unexpected, even irrational, explanation to a reader today. In the nineteenth century, however, this link between sentiment and violent revolutionary politics was frequently made.

Werther's suicide had been presented as evidence of finely cultivated feelings. Nineteenth-century medical writers, however, associated suicide – and, indeed, intense emotion – with mental disease more firmly and unequivocally than anyone had in previous centuries. Psychiatrist Forbes Winslow's *Anatomy of Suicide*, published in 1840, included seemingly randomly selected examples of suicide from remorse, disappointed love, jealousy, wounded vanity, pride, ambition and despair. Rather than showing that someone was a 'man of feeling', suicide was now thought to prove that emotions themselves were abnormal.

Once again, politics came firmly into this idea of normalcy. Winslow reserved particular ire for that 'sect of modern infidels, who falsely denominate themselves *Socialists*'. Robert Owen and his followers were to blame for an increase of suicide in Britain, according to Winslow, because socialism struck 'at the root of all order, and of all virtue, social and public'. Socialists 'break down every barrier of law and restraint, making the passions the only standard of right and wrong – the animal appetites the only test of virtue and vice'.[14] To be led by emotion was abnormal for both the individual and society, according to Winslow, a staunch Conservative. His medical conclusions advanced his political views by drawing on the new politics of emotion that followed the French Revolution. From 1789, reason and emotion became polar opposites, and emotional restraint the defining feature of so-called normal people, conveniently supporting the political status quo.[15]

THE STIFF UPPER LIP

'Are you a "normal person"?' American psychologist (and co-creator of Wonder Woman) William Moulton Marston asked the readers of his book *Emotions of Normal People* in 1928. Most people, Marston concluded, thought they were normal if they did not show frequent extremes of emotion. By the 1920s this view was widespread in psychology and popular thought. While eighteenth- and early nineteenth-century judges wept openly in court, and men and women publicly expressed rage or scorn without being seen as unhinged, this had changed by the beginning of the Victorian era.[16] The teaching of emotional restraint was widespread by 1850, nowhere more so than in British public schools, where a punishing regime was adopted as a way of training boys' bodies and minds to greater endurance.[17] Self-control and self-discipline became the bywords for civilised masculinity, to be inculcated at an early age.

Since emotions emerged in children 'long before the intellect is sufficiently developed or enlightened to direct or control them', Scottish physician Andrew Combe's parental guide, first published in 1840, warned, 'it is obvious that if their proper regulation by the parent be unduly delayed by waiting for the dawn of reason, the character and happiness of the child must remain meanwhile very much at the mercy of accident'.[18] In other words, if parents didn't control children's emotions for them, the child would suffer for it later. American authors had similar advice. Children would quickly exhaust themselves by exhibiting unchecked tears and rages, Henry Clay Trumbull told parents in 1891. Again, the parent had to nip tears and tantrums in the bud, enabling self-control to flourish. Once the child was old enough to understand, he should be 'taught and trained to control his impulse to cry and writhe' and ultimately 'moderate his exhibit of disturbed feeling'.[19]

By the turn of the twentieth century, emotional control had become cast as an ability to put on a brave face to hide one's true feelings, Thomas Dixon explains.[20] First World War propaganda promoted this new ideal to British troops (and nurses), and the British 'stiff upper lip' soon became world-famous. In the 1930s and 1940s it was promoted in the movie theatre through the clipped received pronunciation and no-nonsense manner of film stars like Trevor Howard, Laurence Olivier and James Mason. Of course, their films still made moviegoers cry, even if they tried to hide it. 'I am a very emotional person,' middle-aged housewife Mrs H. told Mass Observation in 1950 when listing the many movies she had cried at. Despite claiming that she was not ashamed of her emotions, Mrs H. 'endeavour[ed] to conceal all traces of emotion in public, except laughter. To cry in public would be like taking off my clothes.'[21] Normal emotion was now private and hidden.

While the Brits tried hard to hide their tears, Americans were busy covering up their anger. In the late nineteenth century, advice manuals and psychological texts emphasised the need for American people to control this emotion in particular. When Marston described the emotions of 'normal people' in 1928, his words were especially damning. 'I do not regard you as a "normal person", emotionally,' he warned, 'when you are suffering from fear, rage, pain, shock, desire to deceive, or any other emotional state whatsoever containing turmoil and conflict.'[22] Marston's model of normal emotions was not necessarily replicated in his personal life. His volatility and petty jealousies were well known to his polyamorous partners, wife Elizabeth Holloway and graduate student Olive Byrne.[23] Nonetheless, the psychologist used emotion to set forth his feminist ideals. The character of Wonder Woman, the original press release stressed, was designed by Marston to 'combat the idea that women are inferior to men, and to inspire girls to self-confidence and achievement in athletics, occupations and professions monopolised by men'. Similarly, *Emotions of Normal People* concluded with a call for women to become the 'love leaders' of the future, overthrowing the 'appetitive' leadership of men and inspiring a general re-education of emotions.[24] Of course, Marston wrote all this while taking credit for his female partners' ideas and work, and dominating the household with his own 'terrifying rages'.[25] Just goes to show, you never can tell what a feminist looks like.

Although Marston went further than most in his desire to promote 'biologically efficient' emotions that produced pleasantness and social harmony, other American psychologists also warned against anger as evidence of 'man's innate destructiveness', as Karl Menninger put it in *Man Against Himself* (1938). For psychoanalyst and popular magazine columnist Dr Karl, this was mostly self-directed anger, a version of Freud's 'death instinct'.[26] Could this rejection of anger be a reaction to the wars of the first half of the century, asked Maryland analyst Frieda Fromm-Reichmann in 1950? 'At the present time,' the Jewish German émigré believed, 'feelings of hostility, antagonism and malevolence between any two individuals seem to be more subject to disapproval in our Western culture, therefore to more repression, than any other unaccept-able brand of human behaviour.'[27] Anger, it seemed, had replaced sex as the human instinct causing the most embar-rassment and disapproval.

Educational films in the 1940s and 1950s pointed out to young Americans how important it was to reign in their frustration and avoid 'emotional loss of control'. They emphasised that 'severe emotional distress often decreases efficiency', making emotional restraint a key measure of individual success as well as family harmony.[28] Lloyd Warner's 1953 book *American Life: Dream and Reality* listed managing anger – alongside sex – as one of the two fun-damental dilemmas of middle-class families when raising children.[29] As in Britain, this view of emotion was class-based: in lower-class America 'rage is freely expressed', Warner believed. Anthropologist Warner no doubt intended to report objectively on differing ways of life. He nonetheless continued the Victorian trend of framing emotion in opposition to reason and intellect by negatively contrasting the 'fist fights' of the working-class teenage boy with the 'initiative, ambition, verbal dexterity and learned economic skills' of his middle-class counterpart.[30]

Anger remained double-edged, however. It increasingly appeared on screen even as it was frowned on in the home. In the 1976 film *Network*, TV news anchor Howard Beale begins to rant uncontrollably on air, only to become more popular than ever before. The movie seems to point to the insecurity and emotionality of the modern media age. 'I'm as mad as hell, and I'm not going to take this any more!' Beale shouts, encouraging ordinary Americans to open their windows and scream his words into the street. At the time *Network* was made, however, ordinary Americans continued to rate anger control as one of the most important personal characteristics.[31] This does not, of course, stop us jumping to conclusions about the 'age of anger' today: even when it turned out to be voters who described themselves as 'dissatisfied but not angry' who were pivotal in Donald Trump's election as American president in 2016.[32]

Today, excessive emotion seems highly visible, from abusive Twitter trolls to recent residents of the White House. But we rarely stop to consider how what we identify as an excess of anger has been shaped by more than 150 years of the glorification of emotional restraint. We also don't consider how specific kinds of emotions may appear more or less abnormal in different cultures. British children have been told for a century or more to repress their tears; Americans to mask their anger. Yet other cultures have different 'rules'. When American anthropologist Jean Briggs spent over a year living with the Utku,* an Inuit group in Northwest Canada, in the early 1960s, her volatile emotions marked her out as a white outsider. She called her account *Never in Anger*, a reflection on what she interpreted as the extreme reserve of the people she lived with. For the Utku, Briggs appeared childish and unsocialised in her emotional reactions. When we, today, try to define a normal level of feeling, our ideas balance somewhere between these two poles: culturally specific, yet weighted down by a history of assumptions about emotion, shaped by attitudes to class, race and gender.

---

* Briggs called the group 'Utku'; their full name is Utkuhikhalingmiut.

PRIMITIVE PASSIONS

One Friday in 1868, eighteen-year-old Belgian seamstress Louise Lateau suddenly began to bleed from her hands and feet. These stigmata were soon accompanied by ecstatic trances, and the Catholic Church, as was their practice, sent a commission to investigate whether or not Lateau's bleeding truly was miraculous. The investigating team included a doctor, Ferdinand Lefebvre, an asylum psychiatrist from Louvain. While Lefebvre initially assumed that the wounds were self-inflicted, he eventually decided that science could not explain Lateau's unusual state.[33] Over the following decade other doctors disagreed, attributing her stigmata to the power they believed the passions had over the body. Strong feelings, they assumed, were especially dangerous to people least able to control their emotions: 'uneducated persons' or those of delicate frame.[34] Once again, this meant women and the working classes.

The ecstasy Lateau experienced, New York physician Meredith Clymer concluded, was 'an emotional disorder characterised by sudden interruption of consciousness and volition'.[35] It was commonly caused by religious enthusiasm, he said, making Louise Lateau's stigmata visible evidence of her disordered emotions. In previous centuries, such strong religious sentiment had been regarded as evidence of piety. Now, American and European doctors attributed Lateau's bleeding to neither miracle nor fraud but to her 'warm imagination', 'delicate frame' and 'excitable temperament'. As a young working-class woman, Louise Lateau was assumed to be especially at risk of disordered feeling.

So too were the 'Hallelujah Lasses' – female officers in the Salvation Army, a new Christian mission founded by William Booth in Britain in 1865. While middle-class women practised charitable and missionary work in other religious contexts, it was only in the Salvation Army that women could preach and give communion, and working-class women at that.[36] The appearance and emotionality of these women was contrasted unfavourably with their prim and proper middle-class counterparts. Eliza Haynes, a girl 'of the roughest factory class', marched through the streets of Nottingham to draw a crowd to a local Salvation Army meeting 'with streamers floating from her hair and jacket, and a placard across her back reading "I am Happy Eliza."' While some were scandalised by Eliza's behaviour, the subsequent meeting was packed. Happy Eliza's advertising clearly worked![37]

Emotions were very much a class affair for the Victorians. The middle classes had self-control – or so they thought – while the masses were emotional and unrestrained. The Salvation Army's public show of enthusiasm 'degraded' the 'national sense of decency' with a religious zeal 'only felt by the stupidest of mankind', the *Saturday Review* bitterly insisted.[38] This idea of abnormal emotion was weaponised. Any exhibition of feeling could be used to discredit someone's views as irrational, while the attribution of excessive feeling to women and working-class people supported their social and political oppression. Lord Curzon, President of the National League for Opposing Woman Suffrage, gave women's lack of 'calmness of temperament' and 'balance of mind' as one of 'fifteen good reasons' for rejecting female suffrage.[39] 'The very temperament of women and the relations of the sexes make voting by women undesirable,' warned American professor Edward Raymond Turner in 1913.[40] It would be irresponsible, the rational elite assured themselves, to give emotionally unstable people the vote.

The idea that strong emotions were 'primitive' was also used to shore up racist beliefs. Just as women might be denied the vote because of their supposed emotional instability, so too did Western scientists justify colonialism through the perceived need for rational rulers. 'The sudden gusts of feeling which men of inferior types display', as evolutionary psychologist Herbert Spencer put it, 'are excessive in degree as they are short in duration'. Some races were of a very 'explosive' nature – like the 'Bushman' (indigenous southern African peoples) – and were thus 'unfit for social union', Spencer declared.[41] Discrediting people through claims about their emotional state – often done by Western scientists who had never actually been to the places about which they were writing – was used to justify oppression.

As in many other efforts to determine a normal standard, this type of thinking was circular. After a lengthy journey around South and West Africa in the 1860s, travel writer William Winwood Reade claimed that the men of the continent were like Western women, with smooth faces and graceful limbs. 'While the women are stupid, sulky and phlegmatic, the men are vivacious, timid, inquisitive, and garrulous beyond belief,' he generalised blithely. African men, Reade said, possessed 'that delicate tact, that intuition, that nervous imagination, that quick perception of character which have become the proverbial characteristics of cultivated women'. This emotional similarity to women made them 'excellent domestic servants'.[42] The supposed emotional differences between white and Black men was used by Reade to validate the colonial hierarchy. If Black men resembled women or children, this 'proved' they were suited to inferior roles. This narrative of 'primitive' emotional states was an important part of the colonial machinery, creating *and* justifying a West-dominated power structure.

Reade himself did not exactly embody the Western rational ideal. He physically attacked local hammock-bearers in Angola after they bumped him against a rock, beating them into 'obsequious bows and deferential smiles'.[43] Served with a bad egg on another occasion, he threw it at the village chief.[44] All the while, Reade saw himself as the white European 'norm' to which every other race was compared. He also considered that he was doing the people of Africa a great service. After all, in his books, Reade railed against the slave trade and determined to 'educate the heart of the Anglo-Saxon people, who are somewhat inclined to pride of colour and prejudice of race'.[45] This only goes to show, of course, that those with progressive political views were not immune from the prejudices embedded in Western norms.

Most European anthropologists and psychologists came to similar conclusions when they compared other races to white European men, again and again reading difference as abnormality. Like Reade, they started with expectations about 'normal' masculine emotions based on the way feelings were expressed in middle-class Europe. Charles Darwin's entry on emotion for *Notes and Queries on Anthropology* – a handbook to help untrained travellers study foreign lands – simply detailed what he expected to find in the West and asked his readers to make a comparison. 'Is extreme fear expressed in the same general manner as with Europeans?' Darwin asked, as if this manner was universal and obvious.[46] 'Apart from kind of feeling,' concluded Spencer, varieties of mankind 'are unlike in amount of feeling'.[47] Black people – like women and the working classes – were impulsive and over-emotional, Spencer and his contemporaries thought. One medical journal, *The Lancet*, suggested that stigmatic Louise Lateau's 'half-hysterical admirers' appeared to 'rival the South Sea savages in the hideous liberties they take with their persons'.[48]

This link – between race, gender and impulsive emotion – lingered in unacknowledged scientific racism for decades, if not centuries. And we can see the legacy of Victorian attitudes in official reactions to passionate political outbursts in Britain, Europe and North America: from the women's suffrage movement of the early twentieth century to the Black civil rights marches of the 1960s. These protests were often characterised by opponents as indicating not the genuine frustrations of participants but the emotionally volatile nature of their sex or race: a dangerous, uncontrolled and unreasonable anger. Bacteriologist Sir Almroth Wright, for example, penned a furious letter to *The Times* in 1912, railing against the 'militant hysteria' in the suffrage movement.[49] 'Suffragettes are variously described by Cabinet Ministers and in leading articles as "maenads", "hysterical young girls", "miserable women" … and so on,' complained Dr Ethel Smyth in response. 'I have never kept such wonderful company as these bright, resolute, indomitable, most normal, and human women.'[50]

This idea of 'militant hysteria' is a charge sometimes

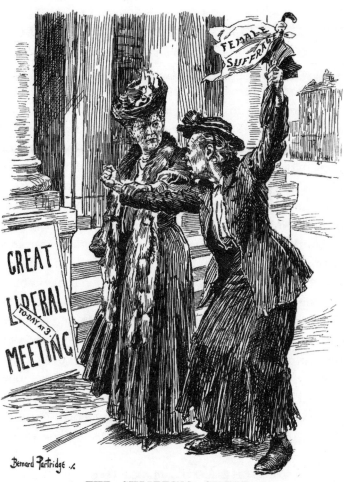

Bernard Partridge .

THE SHRIEKING SISTER.

THE SENSIBLE WOMAN. *"YOU HELP OUR CAUSE? WHY, YOU'RE ITS WORST ENEMY!"*

Cartoon by Bernard Partridge for *Punch* magazine in 1906, making a distinction between the 'emotional' suffragette and the 'sensible' woman.

levelled at young people today, even if the language used has changed. Donald Trump, not exactly known for his calm persona, famously suggested that teenage climate activist Greta Thunberg should 'work on her anger management problem', a suggestion Thunberg turned back on the former president when he tried to contest his election defeat in 2020. Trump has not been alone in trying to use Thunberg's age and gender to discredit arguments he doesn't want to hear. In Britain, right-wing columnist Piers Morgan similarly called Thunberg 'over-emotional'.[51] The toppling of historical monuments associated with the slave trade and the colonial legacies of European countries during Black Lives Matter protests in 2020 were met with similar responses. Young, 'emotional' protesters were simply not allowing the peaceful, rational removal of these statues, critics insisted: even though some statues, like that of Bristol slaver Edward Colston, had been targeted for peaceful removal for decades. Would Colston still be standing in Bristol harbour without the actions of these protesters? Most likely. It's easy enough to be calm and 'rational' when you have all the power (unless you're Donald Trump, perhaps), which is yet another reason why emotional control became an exclusionary tool of the elite.

THE SOUL MACHINE

Although emotional restraint was viewed as an increasingly valuable trait in the Western world during the nineteenth century, it was not something that could be measured. Like most norms, it was an invisible ideal to aspire to. And while notions of 'normal' and 'abnormal' feeling had begun to shape outcomes in European and North American criminal justice systems, the Western obsession with intent and remorse is unusual. Western judges may dispense leniency based on how well defendants perform repentance; in many other cultures, however, what people actually *do* is of primary importance and not the thoughts and feelings underlying or following these actions. Poisoning a village water supply, for example, is a crime of equal seriousness whether it is done intentionally or unintentionally.[52] The arrival of the 'lie detector' emerged from the Western interest in crime and emotional response, turning feeling into something that could be measured and plotted on a graph.

Young Luther Trant, the brilliant but hot-headed assistant to a psychology professor, was an early proponent of such technologies. After the surprise death of a colleague, Trant turned detective, becoming the Sherlock Holmes of experimental psychology. Determined to clear a senior professor's name, Trant performed a range of psychological tests on the suspects. After successfully finding the actual murderer, Trant decided to take a leave of absence from the university to 'try the scientific psychology again', going on to catch killer after killer on the windy streets of early twentieth-century Chicago.[53] Measuring emotion was the secret to Luther Trant's success. It was established 'beyond question', the psychologist-detective insisted, that the resistance of the human body to a weak electric current varied when someone experienced emotion.[54] Trant used a wide variety of devices to record emotion, including the 'soul machine': the 'most delicate and efficient instrument there is for detecting and registering human emotion – such as anxiety, fear, and the sense of guilt'.[55]

Luther Trant was not a real detective. He was the fictional invention of two Chicago journalists, Edwin Balmer and his brother-in-law William MacHarg. But the methods Trant used to measure a level of normal feeling – if not the soul machine itself – were a key feature of twentieth-century study of the emotions. Quantifying emotion was not an easy task. Fifty years before Trant, in 1858, the Utilitarian economist William Stanley Jevons was inspired by reading Quetelet's work on statistics, writing to his sister that he wanted to use mathematics to study society.[56] Emotions, however, stumped him. Jevons was forced to admit that it was 'difficult to conceive' of a 'unit of pleasure or of pain', the two main motivations for human behaviour according to Utilitarian philosophy. This made him 'hesitate to say that men will ever have the means of measuring directly the feelings of the human heart'.[57] Instead Jevons suggested we measure feelings by action.

Another Victorian statistician, Francis Ysidro Edgeworth, went one step further in 1881 by imagining the development of a 'hedonimeter'. This 'psychophysical machine' would continually register 'the height of pleasure experienced by an individual'. Edgeworth poetically described how we find 'the delicate index now flickering with the flutter of the passions, now steadied by intellectual activity, low sunk whole hours in the neighbourhood of zero, or momentarily springing up towards infinity'.[58] Like Trant's soul machine, Edgeworth's hedonimeter never actually existed. However, his description of it shows some of the ways in which Victorian scientists understood passion or emotion: constantly fluctuating, opposed to but potentially controlled by intellect, often barely present at all but occasionally extreme.

In the absence of a hedonimeter, Victorians measured feelings by behaviour and expression, such as blushing – the 'most peculiar and the most human of all expressions', as Darwin put it.[59] Criminals, it was thought, did not blush, which was evidence of their abnormal state. Cesare Lombroso, Italian father of criminology, tested fifty-nine young male criminals, and found that almost half did not 'redden in response to our reprimands, to reminders of their crimes, or to being fixed with a stare, in contrast with normal individuals'. In women, 81 per cent of Lombroso's sample failed to blush when reprimanded, although they did redden when asked about menstrual disorders.[60] For Lombroso, this proved the lack of finer feeling in unrepentant criminals.

In the twentieth century, the fictional hedonimeter became a real-life 'emotiograph', an idea imported to Trant's America from Europe. Turn-of-the-century machines were developed for clinical diagnosis, like that invented by British heart surgeon Dr James Mackenzie in 1906 to detect an irregular heartbeat. But it was not long before these machines were claimed to measure not just physiological change but emotional change too. William Moulton Marston was one of many psychologists who invented a 'lie detector' – the forerunner of today's polygraph – for use in criminal investigations. Marston's polygraph measured breathing and blood pressure, as well as electrical conductance of the skin. Changes in these physiological processes were assumed to indicate heightened emotions. For Trant,

Marston and other psychologists of the era, emotion had suddenly become the proof of guilt. This was, of course, the complete opposite of the *lack* of feeling shown by Lombroso's phlegmatic criminals.

Despite this unexplained shift, use of the polygraph was widespread in the American justice system by 1935. Yet no one had proven that it was definitely measuring emotion, or in what way levels of emotion were linked to guilt, or otherwise normal or abnormal. Amid all this uncertainty, terminology also shifted. By the 1930s the 'lie detector' – as it was now widely known – was claimed to measure truth rather than feeling. Refusing to take a test implied a suspect's guilt, while convicted criminals might even have their sentences overturned following a successful lie detector test.[61] When a tavern in Wisconsin was burgled in 1935,

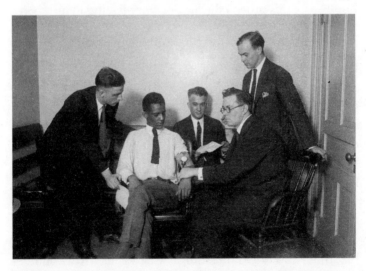

William Moulton Marston (seated on the right) using a polygraph on James Frye in 1922, as part of Frye's appeal against a murder conviction. The appeal was rejected.

bloodhounds quickly led the way to a suspect. The man took a polygraph test and passed, which was assumed to prove his innocence. The bloodhounds were the 'real' liars, it was decided, and the suspect released.[62]

The beauty of these allegedly scientific methods of defining and measuring emotion was that they seemed to be universal. But the polygraph was based on a pre-existing idea of 'normal' emotional reactions. While a test might set a baseline from an individual's specific reaction level, many assumptions were made: that certain physiological reactions are connected to strong emotion, and that a change in these levels means someone is dissembling or guilty. When we try to judge if someone is lying in everyday life, we may simply be reading cultural difference as 'abnormal' behaviour, as one study of American and Jordanian students found.[63] Yet there has been remarkably little attention paid to explaining this link between emotion and reaction, or exploring differences based on culture and upbringing, even if, on occasion, culturally specific 'lie detectors' have been created.[64]

The polygraph itself may also create the distress it measures in its subjects. When, in 2018, Christine Blasey Ford agreed to a polygraph test to support her accusations of sexual assault against Supreme Court nominee Brett Kavanaugh, she described the exam as 'extremely stressful' and recalled crying during testing. By then, the polygraph had come to mean whatever you want it to. Blasey Ford's supporters argued that the results proved her credibility. Her detractors simply claimed that the psychology professor knew how to 'get around' the machine. Measuring our emotions remains extremely contentious. Tests may only prove what we think we already know, a dangerous situation given that these very assumptions are based on cultural expectation and remain influenced by the assumptions embedded in the tests themselves. Despite such huge questions around what, exactly, they measure, polygraphs remain one of the most high-profile ways in which abnormal emotion is measured today, and thousands of Americans undergo the tests every year.[65]

EMOTIONLESS ANDROIDS

While the polygraph assumes guilt by association with emotional excess, the absence of emotion also has a history of criminal investigation. Sometime in 1879, thirty-six-year-old W.B. – let's call him William, a popular name of the time – was walking home after being released from prison in Kingston, Ontario. Within a short distance of his father's house, the ex-convict spotted a horse grazing in a field. Climbing into the pasture, William tied the horse to a telegraph pole and proceeded to severely mutilate the animal. Witnesses struggled to explain William's strange behaviour, which took him immediately back to court, less than a day after he'd been released from a ten-year sentence.

William was born in Swansea, Wales, but his family emigrated to Canada when he was ten years old. According to his stepmother, young William B. had always been of sullen disposition – 'uncommunicative, idle, sly and treacherous' – with a tendency to torture animals and mistreat his younger siblings. Horses were never safe in the neighbourhood, often found with wounded throats where he had slashed them. In 1869, the young man was imprisoned for life for indecently assaulting a ten-year-old girl but mysteriously pardoned and released, taking us back to that day he mutilated a horse on his way home.

William's behaviour was so puzzling that it seemed to the courts that he must be insane. He was acquitted and transferred to the Kingston Asylum. He was still there in 1884, when British psychiatrist Daniel Hack Tuke visited Ontario. Tuke was so fascinated by William that he spent a day reading his case notes and then wrote the whole thing up for a British psychiatric journal. William, Tuke thought, was a classic example of 'moral insanity', with a distinctive twist: his was a *mania sanguinis*, an obsessive thirst for blood.[66]

The diagnosis of moral insanity was introduced by psychiatrist and anthropologist James Cowles Prichard in 1835. Prichard used it to describe people who, without any apparent intellectual impairment or appreciable reason, behaved outside the bounds of convention. Moral here meant psychological or emotional, without necessarily having the ethical connotations we attribute to the term today. The morally insane had weakened 'moral sentiments', an absence of social feeling. This didn't mean they had no emotions at all. Indeed, their lack of social feeling could lead to impulsive outbursts.

When the Victorians spoke of lack of feeling, then, what they generally meant was the absence of a *certain type* of feeling. If a person went against social convention, then he or she must be uncivilised. Tuke concluded that William had reverted to 'an old savage type' and was 'born by accident in the wrong century'. Like so much of Victorian scientific thought, this was supported by racist assumptions. William, Tuke said, 'would have had sufficient scope for his bloodthirsty propensities and been in harmony with his environment, in a barbaric age, or at the present day in certain parts of Africa, but he cannot be tolerated now as a member of civilized society'.[67] The pinnacle of feeling was sympathy and altruism, and, conveniently, white Western men had more of it than anyone else, according to scientists of the time.

Tuke certainly wouldn't have used the term psychopath, not least because he assumed psychopathy to be a type of treatment, like osteopathy or homeopathy.[68] Today, we might think psychopathy describes William's inexplicably vicious acts quite well. While occasionally quiet and useful, he could never be entirely trusted, and it was 'very doubtful if he entertained much affection for anyone'.[69] But what of a jealous young lady or two troublesome five-year-olds who were also morally insane? Or bored gentlewoman Miss M., who sent odd, vaguely threatening letters and the occasional bad drawing of a coffin to young men of her acquaintance? Or Mr C., a civil engineer and 'inventive genius', who travelled by train without buying a ticket?[70] They were all diagnosed with moral insanity, but would you think them psychopaths too?

The term psychopath did not come into scientific use until the twentieth century, and even then it meant something quite different from today. British doctor Albert Wilson was one of the first to publish a scientific analysis of the 'psychopath or human degenerate' – a type of criminal – in 1910. While plenty of late Victorian writers had explored criminal psychology, Wilson described a particular kind of 'unfinished man'. Wilson's psychopath was not the Professor Moriarty or Lex Luther of popular fiction: intelligent 'expert criminals' fell well outside his remit.[71] Instead, the psychopath lay in the 'vast area where we find those who are unable to be classified as normals', well below the 'broad, middle average of intellect and morality, which we all hope to be included in'.[72] These 'sub-normals' were weak-willed, had poor memory and no self-control. Their 'brain architecture', Wilson claimed, was unfinished, meaning they could never hope to become normal. They were not quite 'idiots and imbeciles' – who, he thought, were 'wrecked from birth' – but a new group, 'allied to that class called feeble-minded by the Royal Commission and the College of Physicians'.[73]

Three years later, the Mental Deficiency Act of 1913 enshrined this new category of 'feeble-minded' people in law, imposing restrictions on the lives of people with learning disabilities, unmarried mothers, petty criminals, people living in poverty and others deemed socially undesirable. These were the first 'psychopaths'. Racism once again played a considerable role in defining feeble-mindedness. Wilson concluded – based on 'brain studies' – that his so-called psychopaths were 'a reversion' to the 'negroids and

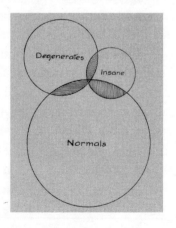

A chart from Wilson's *Unfinished Man* (1910), which aimed to show that the 'three classes' of people were not clearly defined, and 'a few normals of low grade are on the borderline'.

primitive races'.[74] Of course these brain studies, as biologist Stephen Jay Gould has described, had been carried out by white Western scientists, who often performed startling manipulations on their data to prove their assumptions: white men had the biggest – and therefore best – brains.[75]

While there were clear differences between the two categories, the morally insane of the Victorian era and the psychopaths of the Edwardian period shared two characteristics. They were both seen as evidence of 'racial degeneration', and both terms were applied to a wide range of people who flouted convention. These people were not, by any means, what we tend to mean by the term 'psychopath' today: a ruthless, unfeeling individual. Nowadays we might think of a serial killer or a despotic political leader. Until about 1940, however, psychopath meant a huge range of different things. It was sometimes used to describe a tendency towards violent or criminal behaviour. Sometimes it was a synonym for learning disabilities. And sometimes it might be another word for unusual psychological states, like psychosis. It was, says historian Susanna Shapland, something of a 'wastebasket' term, for those deemed not quite mentally 'normal'.[76]

After the Second World War, the psychopath became more clearly defined but also – surprisingly – harder to spot. Take Andrew Lewis, the resident 'psychopath' in a 1960 British Ministry of Health film on understanding aggression. Despite being a difficult customer, Andrew is practised at getting his own way. 'Andrew's stock in trade is his charm, which he can lay on with a trowel whenever it suits him,' his nurse, Henry, complains as Andrew flirts with a female nurse at the hospital cricket match. Unlike the bedraggled, confused female patient in the film, whose violence is seen by nurses as an understandable reaction to her terrifying hallucinations, Andrew is young, well dressed and good-looking. He appears, for want of a better word, *normal*.[77]

Andrew, we are told, was unloved and unwanted even as a baby. By the age of five, 'in this unloved little boy, the ability to love had been stifled'. The character of Andrew Lewis reflects the social view of health popular in Britain after the Second World War, with the new welfare state emphasising social support above individual gain. Those who struggled to display normal emotions were to be pitied and helped, not vilified. Psychopaths are a 'group of struggling humanity, social misfits if you like, who are urgently in need of help', said psychiatrist David Henderson.[78] Henderson laid stress on the impact of negative childhood experiences, which blunted the psychopath emotionally. His work continued, however, to draw on a racist hierarchy of evolution. The psychopath, he said, remained at the emotional level of a 'primitive savage', a Victorian trope still going strong even in 1939.[79]

The leading US expert on psychopathy, Hervey Cleckley, was more critical. He thought that blaming parents or society simply let those who behaved badly off the hook. Besides which, psychopaths were far too widespread for this to be true. Psychopath-finder General Cleckley claimed to have found them everywhere by 1941 – in hospitals, outpatient clinics and in his consultation work. And he was able to help the rest of us spot the psychopaths around us by putting together a handy checklist of psychopathic traits. Cleckley's list of sixteen defining features has profoundly shaped subsequent assessments of psychopathy. Psychopaths, Cleckley declared, were superficially charming and intelligent, unreliable and insincere, and had an 'emotional poverty': a complete absence of 'mature, wholehearted anger, true or consistent indignation, honest, solid grief, sustaining pride, deep joy, and genuine despair'.[80] They did experience joy, anger, despair and so on, but not in the same sustained, mature or genuine way as 'normal' people. Which seems, to someone less well versed in psychopath-spotting than Cleckley, a near impossible thing to measure.

Like Kevin Khatchadourian in *We Need to Talk About Kevin* (Lionel Shriver, 2003), psychopaths in the popular mind today have come to be associated with extreme crime and are largely considered incurable. Yet, while psychopaths in literature and film are almost all serial killers, some psychologists like Robert Hare claim that these 'emotionless androids' are actually all around us.[81] Hare somehow managed to calculate that there are 2 or 3 million psychopaths in North America. Many don't even know they're psychopaths. For the first fifty-eight years of his life, neuroscientist James Fallon thought he was a 'regular guy'. He just happened to be researching the brain scans of psychopaths when he was astounded to find that his own comparative scan showed striking similarities to those of murderers. Fallon's entire philosophy of life – and understanding of neuroscience – was turned on its head by this discovery. He had previously believed that such scans were a straightforward way of understanding human nature, and that our brains and biology account for 80 per cent of who we are. That day, in 2005, Fallon became 'walking, talking proof against my lifelong theory that we are hard-wired to be who we are'.[82]

Yet Fallon's discovery also suggests that the category of 'psychopath' remains less definite and measurable than we might want it to be. Can a brain scan really 'prove' someone to be one? If they never commit a crime, are they indeed a psychopath? Are cold, unfeeling monsters really running most of our businesses, our banks and our governments, as Bob Hare might claim? When you put it that way the whole thing begins to sound like a conspiracy theory: the invasion of the psychopathic body snatchers writ large. The more we hear about psychopaths, the more we see them around us. That's what happened to Jon Ronson while he was writing *The Psychopath Test*, after all.[83] Or perhaps it's the other way around. We hear about something terrible that someone has done, and we look for explanations in their behaviour and expressions. Do they feel like we feel? Or are they one of the androids Hare described, unable to understand what 'real humans' experience?

Science fiction has popularised the android comparison. Take Lieutenant Commander Data, who appeared in *Star Trek: The Next Generation* from 1987, searching for and over-thinking human emotional experience for the next fifteen years. The empathy tests in Philip K. Dick's *Do Androids Dream of Electric Sheep?* were similarly used to identify non-human replicants. Yet the humans in Dick's 1968 novel also manipulate their emotions, programming themselves with a 'mood organ' to experience anything from greater ire to win an argument to scheduling in a 'six-hour self-accusatory depression'.[84] Who can say what is more genuine? The engineered replicants or the programmed humans?

Anyway, much to Hare's annoyance, we remain more likely to relate lack of feeling to specific acts and crimes. This makes us feel safer, perhaps – who needs an expensive Bob Hare course if we can spot a killer by their cold dead eyes? But how often are we led by our assumptions? In 2012, for example, twelve people were murdered in a cinema in a Denver suburb by former neuroscience student James Holmes, who opened fire during a screening of *Batman: The Dark Knight Rises*. When video footage of Holmes at his arraignment was shown on TV, one of my friends commented on his cold, emotionless expression. To her, he looked like a psychopathic killer. To me, he simply looked heavily medicated.

This reminds us that showing emotion is not always easy. A colleague once told me about her brother's experience after being diagnosed with schizophrenia. He was mostly okay on his medication, she said, though he often complained that he was numb and couldn't feel anything at all. When their mother died, he stopped taking anti-psychotics for a week. It would be wrong, he told his sister, to go to his mother's funeral and be unable to cry. She didn't dispute this. The way we read the emotions of others is shaped by our understanding of a situation just as much as cultural difference and individual variation, and sometimes the added complication of drugs or alcohol. We might rush to judgement or struggle to pick up on emotional cues. This can be harder for some neurodivergent people, but I would be surprised if there's anyone who cannot think of a time when they have misunderstood someone else's feelings. Whether it's about the expectations of others or our own assumptions about right and wrong, normal and abnormal, the messy uncertainty of emotion is often what makes us feel human.

LIVING WITH FEELING

Just before my thirtieth birthday, I got a job in a historic house museum. I was excited about my new role. I loved the fact that when I came to work in the morning, I had the key to the front door of a Georgian townhouse, letting myself in as if I lived there. I loved the way the stairs slanted and the dark rooms smelled of polished wood. One day, I showed a middle-aged American woman round the building; she was interested in hiring the museum for a corporate event. I cheerfully told her about the history, taking her from room to room as I shared my love of the house and its past. As we reached the top floor and I paused for breath, she looked at me sternly. 'You're *very* enthusiastic!' she said darkly.

I never learned exactly what it was that this stranger thought was so excessive about my enthusiasm. But many of us today do retain a certain suspicion of heightened emotion, especially, perhaps, in strangers. In Poland, smiling at a stranger is considered abnormal – as I learned the hard way on a visit to Kraków, when my automatic grins at dour shop assistants were met with bewilderment. Emotions are something to be closely guarded, admitted only to a chosen few. And sometimes the British are just as concerned by falsity: the cheesiness of the casual 'Have a great day!' As a nation, we're still living with the historical emotional hangover of the 'stiff upper lip' – even if, more recently, concerns with emotional honesty or being 'true' to ourselves have begun to emerge.

Where does this leave us? What are the emotions of normal people? Should we reject all negative feeling, and embrace love and understanding to become the Wonder Women of the future? Or is repressing grief and anger dangerous in itself – as Sigmund Freud and his circle came to believe? More recently, the concept of 'emotional intelligence', popularised by psychologist Daniel Goleman in 1995, has come to the fore. In this model, often known as EQ, emotions are not so much internal desires, to be regulated or released by an individual, but understood in terms of a 'capacity' for relationships with others. Yet novels, television shows and films continue to emphasise the challenges this complicated history has brought us. Emotional honesty either appears an impossible ideal or something to be mocked, a needy desire for attention, like the troubled Tanya McQuoid in the HBO comedy-drama *The White Lotus* (2021).

A century of emotiographs and soul machines has, after all, brought us no closer to measuring the intensity of our feeling; or even finding a universal way of describing or understanding emotion. In 1971, psychologist Paul Ekman began to argue for a set of fundamental emotional expressions and so-called 'basic' emotions across all cultures. Ekman's model has had widespread influence, even appearing in the 2015 Disney/Pixar film *Inside Out*. The number of emotions in Ekman's model have changed over time, but it usually includes anger, disgust, fear, happiness, sadness and surprise (the last perhaps too vague for the cartoon world and thus unceremoniously dropped by

Disney). Yet these 'basic' emotions, and the expression of them, are not as universal as Ekman first assumed. One study found that people living in remote islands in Papua New Guinea interpret the Western 'fear' face as angry and threatening.[85] And how often do any of us feel simple, discrete emotions in response to everyday life anyway? As a 2021 study using emotional expressions made by professional actors concluded, 'facial movements and perceptions of emotion vary by situation and transcend stereotypes of emotional expressions'.[86]

When definitions of normal feeling are created with a particular group in mind, they can become a self-fulfilling prophecy. The emotional restraint or specific expressions of feeling prevailing in one group can become the way others are judged and measured. Over the last two centuries, this has often been used as an argument for supporting the status quo. An elitist, racist science of feeling proposed that the people with the most political and economic power in the nineteenth and twentieth centuries were simply the best people – those with the finest social feeling. Their subjugation of others – through colonialism, sexism or class-based repression – was presented as the act of a benevolent parent, who knows what is best for their child's emotional and physical well-being. Some of the negative stereotypes associated with these assumptions have lingered in the popular imagination, from the angry young Black man to the emotionally manipulative woman. We might assume that our emotions are hardwired into human nature, a fundamental part of who we are. The history of emotions, however, shows us how these norms have themselves been constructed – and to whose benefit, or detriment.

6

ARE MY KIDS NORMAL?

When I was three years old, I told the teachers at playgroup that my toys came alive at night. My teddies and I flew to Otford Palace in Kent to have dinner with my best friend, King Henry VIII. I drew them a picture to prove it. No one batted an eyelid at my night-time visits to a long-dead Tudor king. But, a few miles away at another playgroup, my friend Sophie had quite a different experience when she told her teachers she was a little cat. 'Don't play with the scissors, Sophie,' they warned her, and she cast them a withering glance. 'Cats don't understand English!' she said scornfully. Worried that Sophie's behaviour wasn't normal, the teachers called her parents. 'Do you think she might need to see a psychiatrist?' they said. 'Perhaps she really *does* think she's a cat!' She didn't.

The ways children grow and develop, the way they act and the things they do, have proved some of the most emotive and contentious ways of placing limits on normal behaviour in the last two centuries. We worry about the normal weight and development of infants, whether or not our children are learning or socialising properly, and if their behaviour or emotions are problematic. The Victorians were more concerned than their forebears about normal childhood: children were no longer conceived of as tiny adults but had specific needs through childhood and adolescence to shape them into ideal citizens. The introduction of compulsory schooling, the passing of child labour laws, and the raising of the age of consent in 1885 were all part of a new desire to protect and reform the child, an impetus that continued into the twentieth century, becoming particularly acute in the last fifty or so years.

These fears said as much about adults as they did about children: 'They fuck you up, your mum and dad,' as Philip Larkin put it.[1] While the misanthropic poet's final advice was not to have kids at all, large numbers of us don't heed this warning. We do, however, take on board Larkin's fears about handing our oddities to our offspring. The Victorians feared the 'tyranny of organisation' which meant, they believed, that children born to neurotic parents were fated to follow in their footsteps. The psychiatrist who invented this phrase, Henry Maudsley, certainly didn't have kids of his own. As the twentieth century turned, parenting began to rise up the agenda. No longer was caring for children something instinctual and natural, but a skill that needed to be learned: first, in the early decades of the century, focusing on the physical health of the infant and later, around the Second World War, the child's emotional needs. By this time the concern was less that a parent might infect their child with unstable genetics, but that at every step of development they might fail their offspring.

My own parents certainly worried about this. When I

was a teenager, my mum apologised to me. 'Neither your father nor I are very good at dealing with other people,' she admitted. 'I think we've passed it on to you; I'm sorry.' While she might have thought of this as an admission of failure, it was significant to me as an awkward, confused teen. It certainly made me feel less alone. And, although her words could have encouraged a sense of fatalism – 'if my parents are like this too, I can't ever change' – it didn't. It made me determined to learn to manage social situations better. Despite finding human contact intensely uncomfortable, I trained myself to accept hugs. It took years but today, not only can I hug a friend without flinching, but I do it without even thinking. It might not sound like a big deal. To me, it was massive.

Childhood development is not set in stone. Children invariably have the capacity to astonish and move us with their ideas and insight. They might surprise us by the ways in which their feelings and behaviour differ from our own; or when we compare them to a category we've been told they fit into. They can also frequently impress or interest us when we compare them to their peers. Amid these myriad differences, how do we understand and define normal childhood development? And when does it help or hinder a child to be labelled abnormal? From first steps to first dates, we compare our children's lives to a set of standards as we worry that we as parents, as much as they as children, may be shown to come up lacking.

THE FAT, HEALTHY BABY

My first niece was born in 2017. She was a healthy and happy baby, who slept and ate well, and was much doted on by an excited family. She was also relatively small. When her weight was plotted on a chart, she always fell between the 50th and the 25th percentile (meaning that fifty to seventy-five babies in every 100 were bigger than her). 'Everyone always praised big babies,' my sister remembers, 'saying, "Ooh, mummy's milk is great!" It's always well-meaning, but it makes you feel bad to have a smaller baby, even though by definition half the babies are under 50 per cent.' She recalls one time when she took her new baby to a weigh-in, and the health visitor frowned: 'She's on the 30 per cent line, hmm. Come back next week and we'll keep an eye on her.' My sister went away anxious, determined to feed the baby more and increase her weight. But when she went back the next week, another health visitor had a different view. 'Great! She's in the 28th percentile and bang on track on the same line since the start. She looks perfect!' The figure had barely changed, it had simply been interpreted differently. My sister shakes her head, sighing. 'So, I had worried for a week for nothing, just based on a chart.' It took her a while to be comfortable with her baby's size, and even longer to feel confident that everyone around her also thought the baby was fine.

One of the earliest things we measure in our children is growth. Are they growing properly, or getting enough nourishment? Although we are constantly bombarded with the message that breastfeeding is the most important thing for a new baby's health, it's usual for mothers to have difficulty with it. One US study of 418 new mothers found that 92 per cent reported problems with breastfeeding in the first few days after giving birth. Sometimes this was difficulty getting the baby to settle or latch on to the breast, sometimes a lack of milk or an excess of pain. These issues were not always resolved; two months later, nearly a quarter of women in the study had given up breastfeeding altogether.[2] This isn't just a modern issue, of course. Writer Vera Brittain tried and failed to breastfeed her first baby, born in 1927, and blamed a lack of support from professionals, just as some women today do.[3]

In Vera Brittain's time, mothers were judged even more harshly on the size of their babies. In 1906 George Newman, London Medical Officer of Health for Finsbury, declared that 'infant mortality is a social problem'. Birth rates had been falling in England and Wales since 1881 but infant mortality had not declined at the same rate. In 1899, 163 children in every thousand died before they reached their first birthday, greater than the average across the rest of the decade.[4] Mortality rates were higher in poorer districts, like Newman's area of London. However, Newman did not conclude that infant mortality was caused by poverty. Instead, he called it an 'an indication of the existence of evil conditions in the homes of the people' and 'in some way intimately related to the social life' of the country.[5] Infant mortality said more about mothers than it did about babies, according to Newman, for 'expressed bluntly, it is the ignorance and carelessness of mothers that directly causes a large proportion of the infant mortality'.[6]

Newman and his colleagues concluded that lack of breastfeeding and the use of diluted tinned milk were

to blame. This conveniently sidestepped the wider issue
that many women were themselves too malnourished
to provide adequate milk for their babies, and buying
decent milk was far too expensive for most working-class
families.[7] The emphasis on feeding also meant that the
increasing size of an infant became newly emphasised as
a widespread measure of health. The routine weighing of
babies had begun in Germany in 1878.[8] By the 1890s, it
was accepted practice by doctors across Europe and North
America. It was the health visitor, however, who took this
into British homes in the early twentieth century. In 1905,
fifty towns across England and Wales were employing paid
health visitors and in 1907 it became law that all births
must be notified within six weeks to enable a health visitor
to attend.[9]

Health visitors were expected to advise working-class
mothers and measure the condition of the children they
visited. Greta Allen's 1905 *Practical Hints to Health Visitors*
offered two ways to identify a normal, healthy baby: by
weight, and by the colour and consistency of stools ('beat-
en-up eggs' were okay; 'chopped spinach' a worry).[10]
Several decades of baby weighing as medical practice
meant that 'normal' weight could be defined by averages.
Allen thus published a handy weight table that health visitors could use for comparison, giving the normal weight
and height of a child from birth to the age of fifteen. The
origin of the figures, reproduced from a book by a New
York doctor, was rather vague; they were averages 'from
original sources, and are drawn from about 500 cases'.[11]
Were these 500 mystery infants and toddlers healthy and
well-fed? We are not told the answers to this question and

yet the average weight of these babies becomes an exact definition of normal infant health, shorn of any context.

When weight charts define a baby's health it's easy to forget that – by the law of averages – some babies will be smaller than others. At infant welfare clinics in the 1900s, weight cards had to be completed for every attending infant.[12] These clinics also used exact figures as the comparative normal weight at each age (usually based on an average), making it almost impossible for real babies to measure up. Advice was easy to give and harder to follow. One 'girl-mother' at the St Pancras School for Mothers, opened in 1907, sobbed when told her baby had lost weight despite 'struggling with all the odds against her to follow out the instructions given her to the very letter'.[13]

Busy mothers – poor and rich alike – became a target for the medical profession. One middle-class mother was told by her doctor that she 'was probably dashing about too much and "churning" my milk and taking the goodness away'.[14] Working mothers, meanwhile, were the cause of 'verminous children' with lice or fleas, warned Enid Eve, Chief Health Visitor and Sanitary Inspector in central London.[15] The health visitor 'should do everything in her power to render crèches unnecessary by persuading mothers to stay at home with their children', Eve insisted.[16] This became a running theme in child guidance until well after the Second World War. The London Medical Officers of Health were especially concerned by malnourishment when 'the mother goes to work and is unable to provide a proper midday meal for her children', even though three times as many underweight children were living in poverty as those reported as neglected by parents.[17]

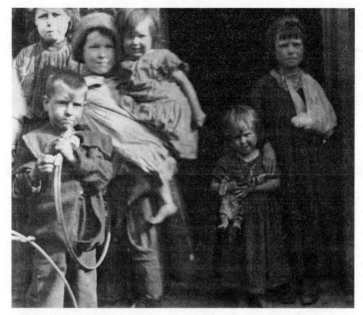

Photograph of children living in poverty in London's East End, c.1900.

Some reformers were more insistent about the effects of poverty and the environment on children's development. From 1909 to 1913 the Fabian Women's Group, led by Australian-born socialist and feminist Maud Pember Reeves, surveyed forty-two low-income families in Lambeth, South London. They published the results as *Round About a Pound a Week*: the average wage of participants in the study (20 shillings). Some politicians who argued that poverty – and thus child malnutrition – was caused by recklessness claimed that any family could survive on a pound a week. The families Reeves studied, however, had to budget very carefully on this income. Every saving might have effects on the family's health. One good, airy upstairs room, Reeves found, could cost as much in rent as several damp basement rooms, leaving families to juggle overcrowding against unsanitary living conditions. Infant mortality rose as the amount spent on rent decreased.[18]

'There is no doubt', Reeves solemnly declared, 'that the healthy infant at birth is less healthy at three months, less healthy still at a year, and often by the time it is old enough to go to school it has developed rickets or lung trouble through entirely preventable causes.'[19] She described some of these children in moving detail. Emma, aged ten and '4 feet 6 in her socks', was a 'queer little figure, the eldest of six, with a baby always in her arms'. Dorothy, a two-year-old 'ex-baby' was 'devoured with a desire to accompany her elder brothers and sisters to school' and seethed with restlessness and anxiety in a high-chair while her mother managed a new infant. Benny was twelve, small for his age and 'very, very serious'. While his father was out of work, Benny offered to work for the local milkman for two hours before and after school, without telling his parents.[20] Despite their poor housing and inadequate diets, Reeves noted that the children were 'well brought up as regards manners and cleanliness and behaviour' and 'kindly and patiently treated by their mothers'. As the children grew older, however, their most salient feature was 'want of the joy of life'. Like their mothers, these youngsters came to accept the limitations imposed upon them. 'These children never rebel against disappointment,' Reeves concluded. 'It is their lot. They more or less expect it.'[21]

The Fabian Women's Group recommended a minimum wage, child benefit, free school meals and school clinics to support the healthy physical development of children. It would take a long time for these measures to be brought in. After the First World War, poverty remained widespread, worsened by unemployment and depression in the 1930s. But there were changes in the scientific understanding of child health too. Vitamins – or 'accessory food factors' – were newly trumpeted as the key to good health and development in the child. Formula milk was supplemented with fruit juice and Virol (a brand of malt extract) to prevent scurvy and rickets and, in 1928, pharmaceutical company Glaxo began to add vitamin D to its baby-milk formula.[22]

Knowledge of vitamins – the new thing 'everyone has heard of' – seemed to open up a positive new era for child health.[23] The bone deformities caused by rickets, for example, had long been visible among inner-city youngsters. By 1925, the Medical Officer of Health for Walthamstow (in what is now north-east London) claimed that knowledge of vitamins had had a noticeable effect on the health of schoolchildren.[24] This was rather premature. Awareness of vitamins didn't mean they were available to all children. In 1943, the Oxford Nutrition Survey studied the physical and nutritional health of children in three districts, including Walthamstow. Levels of vitamin C were 'well below the accepted optimum level' in Birmingham, Walthamstow and Oxfordshire towns and 'within normal range' only in Oxfordshire villages, where fresh fruit and vegetables were grown. More than 40 per cent of children were found to be in poor health, even when those below normal weight 'but otherwise well' were classed as healthy.[25]

After the Second World War, doctors began to stress the huge range of variation in healthy children. 'Any doctor may be able to say what the average weight and height is for a child of given age and sex,' Professor of Child Health Ronald Illingworth commented in 1953, 'but no one can say what the normal is, for it is impossible to define the normal.'[26] Even if one could define it, the average child was not the same as in earlier decades. In 1959, the Ministry of Health reported that normal weight charts from the 1920s contained lower figures than the averages from 1940s and 1950s studies of babies and children. The survey proposed to update the norms to reflect the fact that infants and children had become 'heavier and taller'.[27] Health officials in the 1950s generally saw this as positive; an increase in average size was a sign of 'better feeding and general care'.[28]

There were dissenting voices, though. Some medical officers of health began to declare that 'overnutrition' and obesity were shortening lives.[29] By the mid-1960s, the now familiar phrase 'childhood obesity' had begun to appear, already cast as an epidemic of dangerous proportions. In 1962, *The Times* reported that local education authorities in Cambridgeshire had responded to the rising weight of children by banning buns and doughnuts in school tuckshops – replacing them with no less fatty potato crisps and salted peanuts.[30] Later that same year, the newspaper declared the 'fine fat baby' to be a fallacy, with the problem of overweight children 'so serious' that poster campaigns in clinics should be used to warn mothers of the danger.[31]

A rise in obesity, according to school medical officer Phyllis Gibbons, was linked to a higher standard of living accompanied by a change in eating habits, and 5–15 per cent of schoolchildren were now 'at least 10 per cent above the mean weight for their age, height and body build'.[32] Of course, it was perfectly possible that this had always been the case in a normal distribution of weight. In the post-war era, however, it was newly presented as a problem. Gibbons described two 1965 experiments with dieting for small groups of teenage girls in Croydon; four years later, her trial had expanded into a 'borough-wide provision of school weight-control clinics'.[33] By the end of the decade, other London boroughs had introduced Weight Watchers schemes targeting 'overweight' teens, usually girls, following on the heels of the first ever Weight Watchers meeting in the UK in 1967. These programmes newly focused on children and teenagers, not just adults as 1930s diets had done.[34]

Thirty years later, governments and health campaigners across the Western world really latched on to the idea of an 'obesity epidemic'. *The Times*, forgetting that it had first laid claim to a crisis in 1962, pointed in 2001 to an 'alarming increase in child obesity'. The article described a study published in the *British Medical Journal*, stating that the number of children judged overweight had gone up by 50 per cent between 1984 and 1994.[35] The statements made were not all that different from the concerns of the late 1960s, with perhaps a little less attention to the breadth of variation. Nonetheless, it seemed to strike a chord, and a 'barrage of consultations and reports addressing obesity', including in children, appeared during 2004, painting a dystopian future.[36] The problem of being overweight was 'transformed from one affecting individuals to one affecting society and nation', just as the issue of the malnourished infant had been in the early 1900s.[37]

It's this that seems to be the unifying factor where the size of the normal child is concerned. The normal child – and, by extension, the normal mother – has for the last century or more been at the centre of political and cultural concerns about the future of the nation. From the underweight and neglected infant of the early 1900s, whose working mother failed in her duty to her country, to the obese and inactive millennial, the normal child highlights fears for the future of society. Worries about malnutrition and childhood obesity reflect concerns about parents, about poverty, gender and class, rather than shedding much light on the normality of any individual child. When we look at a child in the context of their circumstances, they are probably far less abnormal than standards might suggest. If children are judged abnormal in a community, it is usually because there is 'a basic flaw in the community itself', paediatrician Jan van Eys claimed in 1979.[38] The history of the normal child certainly bears out this statement.

THE GENIUS OF EARLSWOOD ASYLUM

James Henry Pullen was fifteen years old when he was admitted to the Royal Earlswood Asylum – or the National Asylum for Idiots, as it was then called. Located on Earlswood Common in Redhill, Surrey, this was the first charitable institution for 'idiot children' in England and Wales. Pullen arrived in 1850, accompanied by classmates from Essex Hall in Colchester, one of a small handful of schools for children with special educational needs. Like these other 'idiot and imbecile children' – as the harsh

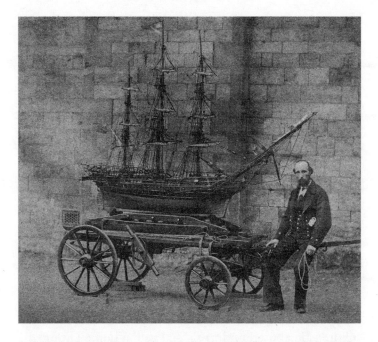

James Henry Pullen, sitting on the end of a wooden trolley upon which one of his model ships rests, photographed by G. E. Shuttleworth, undated (after 1867).

medical language of the Victorian era described them – Pullen had struggled to learn in traditional environments. He developed slowly, not speaking his first word until the age of seven. No school would accept him, and the young Pullen remained at home until the age of twelve, when he was sent to Essex Hall. Here, under the watchful eye of schoolmistress Sarah Pearce, James Henry Pullen learned to spell his first word: 'man'.

At Earlswood, the teenage Pullen entered what would become his permanent home. It was very different from the comfortable three-storey house in Dalston where he had grown up. The vast, imposing edifice was built to house

400 residents: all, at the time of admission, aged between eight and eighteen. These children had to be deemed likely to benefit from the institution, and their families to be 'respectable' working men and women, who had never received Poor Law relief.[39] The 'Idiot' Asylum was a counterpart to the County Lunatic Asylums that were springing up around England and Wales in the 1840s and 1850s, each one a grand architectural showcase of Victorian philanthropy.

Of course, since Pullen's time, attitudes to these institutions have changed remarkably. When Earlswood finally closed in 1997 many people were relieved to see it go, associating institutional life with neglect, abuse and negative attitudes towards people with a learning disability. In 1850, however, the institution was heralded as a sign of a better age. No longer, the founders trumpeted, would these children be abused and neglected in the home (although, according to historian Simon Jarrett, this hadn't actually been widespread before the asylums were built).[40] In the asylum, they would be well fed and housed. They would learn to become useful members of society, trained in domestic skills and manual labour, and taught to interact with others.

That doesn't mean that the children admitted to Earlswood were happy to be there, or even well cared for. Like Pullen, they had no choice about their new home. Sent to Earlswood by family members unable or unwilling to care for them, these young people had been identified as mentally abnormal by parents and doctors alike. Ten-year-old Robert Campbell, said the surgeon who examined him, 'had a "vacant indifference as to objects such as usually attract children and general conduct unlike other children"'.[41] William Green's mother complained that he was unable to read, even though she had spent considerable time trying to teach him.[42]

Pullen continued to struggle with formal learning throughout his teenage years at Earlswood. He could speak few words, and never learned to read and write. Yet he nevertheless became one of Earlswood's most famous residents: the 'genius of Earlswood Asylum' as he was hailed in the press. Since his youth, Pullen had been skilled at sketching and building model ships. At Earlswood, he was introduced to craft training and excelled. Aged twenty, Pullen was given his own workshop and a small wage as the institution's carpenter. He made furniture for the hospital as well as pursuing his own projects: from an impressive scale model of Brunel's SS *Great Eastern* to a mechanical giant that stood outside his workshop. The reason for James Henry Pullen's combination of mechanical brilliance and learning disability remains under debate. In Pullen's time, however, learning disabilities were assumed to be hereditary, perhaps another sign of degeneration.

As in other Victorian classificatory systems, assumptions about heredity were based on racist and racial categories, which divided humans into groups based on physical features. When psychiatrist John Langdon Down, Pullen's doctor, first described the syndrome for which he became famous, it was part of an 'ethnic classification of idiots', as he called it.[43] Many residents of Earlswood, Down claimed, could be 'referred to one of the great divisions of the human family other than the class from which they have sprung'. Although all were of white European heritage,

Down declared that in their features he had found, among other examples, 'specimens of white negroes', 'types of the family which people the South Sea islands', and the so-called 'Mongolian type of idiocy'. This last was the first description of the syndrome that would be named after him: Down's Syndrome.[44] The 'racial' features Down claimed to have observed were, he said, evidence of atavism: a reversion to a primitive state. They were also yet more evidence of the way 'abnormal' for many white Victorians meant non-Western; Down's classifications discriminated against people of colour as well as people with a learning disability.

It wasn't only scientific classification that altered the way certain children were understood; so too did the rise in formal education.[45] To put it simply, as increasing numbers of the population learned to read and write, those who struggled to do so – like William Green and James Henry Pullen – became more visible, and at an earlier age. It was in the classroom that the idea of normal intelligence in children was most clearly defined. In England and Wales, school attendance was made compulsory in 1880.[46] At the same time, learning to read and write became more highly valued for both men and women, including those who did not use these skills in their daily work.[47] In 1840, two-thirds of men and half of women in England were literate; by the end of the century, almost three-quarters of both sexes could read and write.[48]

The same occurred across much of Europe: free primary education was made compulsory in France in 1881 and basic literacy was almost universal by the end of the nineteenth century. It was in this context that, in 1904, psychologist

Alfred Binet was asked by the French minister of public education to improve the skills of children who struggled in the classroom. To identify these children, Binet and his research assistant Théodore Simon tried to measure basic processes in learning (as they called them): skills in ordering items, comprehension, invention and correcting mistakes. By using a huge range of different tests, Binet hoped to find a way of identifying each child's learning potential. His tests were not meant to rank *all* children, but to provide greater insight into the abilities of those already struggling. This would enable teachers to provide help and support so that the child's intelligence could be improved.[49] IQ (intelligence quotient), as it later became known, was not at first seen as an inherited, unchanging entity.

It was, however, defined by comparison to the 'normal', unlike previous tests of intelligence that had claimed an absolute result. Today, we are used to the idea that intelligence varies from an average. A hundred and fifty years ago, it was not at all inevitable that this view would take hold, or that a trait called intelligence might fall on a normal distribution. When Francis Galton published *Hereditary Genius* in 1869 – a book which claimed on very little evidence that genius was inherited – Charles Darwin called himself a convert. 'I have always maintained that, excepting fools, men did not differ much in intellect,' Darwin wrote to Galton in December of that year, 'only in zeal & hard work.'[50] After reading Galton's book, Darwin changed his mind. Yet Darwin's previous position was quite reasonable. His own work on evolution had shown what a lengthy process natural selection was. He had argued that humans evolved mentally as a species, not as individuals. If that were true, why should mental faculties vary significantly between people?

Having converted his cousin to the idea that intelligence varied across the population, Galton sought to popularise the idea, and prove that intelligence could be measured on a normal distribution. He plotted the grades obtained by Cambridge students on a bell curve and used this to create a general rule for human intelligence, from 'idiots and imbeciles' at the bottom of the scale to geniuses at the top. By the 'assured law of deviations from an average', Galton confidently declared, human intelligence formed a bell curve, with its peak being the average mental level of humankind.[51] It's largely thanks to this Victorian eugenicist that we now tend to assume intelligence is a fixed inborn trait, which is surely reason enough to pause to reconsider the notion.

But back to Alfred Binet. His tests were also stan-dardised on 'normal' children, including Binet's own. They carried out a range of tasks which were assigned an age by which most children managed to complete them. A normal child of four should, according to Binet, be able to give their sex, name basic objects, repeat three numbers and compare two lines of different length. A child of seven could point to their right hand and left ear, describe a picture and name four colours. By age ten, a child could arrange five weights in order, copy drawings from memory, criticise absurd statements and understand difficult ques-tions.[52] Presumably Binet also thought that children at this age were rather morbid: most of his 'absurd statements' involved terrible accidents or grievous bodily harm. 'The body of an unfortunate young girl, cut into eighteen pieces, was found yesterday on the fortifications,' began one particularly unpleasant example; 'it is thought that she killed herself.' The correct response was that the poor girl would not have been able to cut herself into eighteen pieces.[53] Whether or not Binet's participants had nightmares after his tests was not recorded.

What of those children who could not complete all the tasks assigned to their age? These slower developers were divided into three groups, all labelled with scientific names that quickly entered common use as insults. Children who could pass only the tests for one- and two-year-olds – assuming their actual age was higher – were 'idiots'. Those with the abilities of three- to seven-year-olds were 'imbeciles'. The 'moron' fell anywhere between eight and twelve years on Binet's scale. Four years later, a German psychologist named William Stern tweaked Binet's scale by dividing the child's mental age by their chronological age. This number, expressed as a percentage, formed the so-called intelligence quotient (IQ).[54] An IQ of 100 was the norm not because it was necessarily the average of the population – Binet's tests did not measure an average but the capacity of 'most' children – but because it expressed the

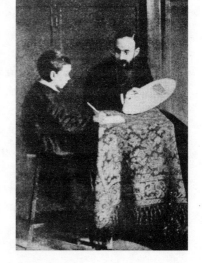

Photograph of Alfred Binet carrying out a test on a child, by an anonymous photographer, 1907.

idea that the mental and physical age of the child were equal. A mental age of 12 divided by a chronological age of 12 came to 1 – or 100 per cent.

When Binet's tests were imported to the US, however, they were newly used to rank *everyone*, not just children. American psychologists assumed that intelligence test scores were linked to social status. The social hierarchy, according to psychologist Lewis Terman, designer of the Stanford–Binet IQ test, was simply 'common sense'.[55] But what is common sense other than seeing things as they happen to be? The privileged conditions that the elite were born into, and the opportunities wealthy parents could give their children, ensured that it was easy for Francis Galton's geniuses to be replicated. Early twentieth-century intelligence testers saw the status quo reflected back at them and assumed it was a product of nature.

Not only this, but many of their tests were biased. This could be because their questions were culturally specific; for example: 'Crisco is a: patent medicine; disinfectant; toothpaste; food product?' – would you know the answer without looking it up? The bias could be because a topic was most familiar to a certain class – did everyone have the means to purchase Crisco? Or it might be because questions presented a certain model of society – one that privileged consumerism and brand identification.* If what we are testing is whether or not children have a white, Western, middle-class lifestyle, then the 1917 Army Alpha IQ test – the exam that sparked a thousand others, and from which the above question about Crisco comes – is a

---

* It's a food product (used for baking). Did you guess right? Probably, if you have spent a lot of time in North America. Probably not if you haven't.

very good measure. If we are claiming the test measures a specific trait within the psychology of the individual, it is less useful. Nonetheless, these tests were used to determine, among other things, immigration quotas, job roles and a child's educational path.

But perhaps the most bizarre thing about IQ – a supposedly fixed, inherited characteristic – is how the measurements themselves have changed over the years. IQ tests have been 're-normed' continuously since 1932 to make sure that 100 remained at the centre of the bell curve. If you took a 1932 test and a 1947 test at the same time, you would get a higher IQ score from the earlier test. Psychologist James Flynn pointed out in 1984 that the total gain in American subjects over forty-six years amounted to an increase of an incredible 13.8 IQ points, replicated in studies across many other countries.[56] Were people getting cleverer? Were they getting more used to standardised tests? Or was it something else entirely? Flynn came to the conclusion that IQ tests could only be loosely associated with intelligence.

IQ testing did not die with this realisation. It continued to be used to support class, race and social prejudices, as in psychologist Richard Herrnstein and political scientist Charles Murray's controversial 1994 volume *The Bell Curve*. Like their Victorian predecessors, Herrnstein and Murray regarded the normal distribution as evidence of genetic differences in intelligence between races and social classes. 'Scholars accept' that 40–80 per cent of IQ is genetically inheritable, the pair blithely and wrongly claimed.[57] If those with more wealth and education tend to have higher IQ, then this proved, Herrnstein and Murray thought, that superior intelligence had found its rightful place. Yet again, the bell curve provided a convenient way of supporting pre-existing prejudice.

What has a century of IQ tests proved, then? Are we born with a fixed intelligence, which can be measured when we are children and which remains unchanged throughout our lives? Or does intelligence vary little between people, as Charles Darwin once thought? Psychologists today are increasingly critical of IQ testing, even if many still hold to the idea that intelligence exists and can be measured. There remain far more questions than answers about what normal intelligence could or should be.[58] And, as funding for special educational needs and disabilities (SEND) facilities decreases across the UK, Binet's aim of using testing to determine the support needs for an individual child seems like a distant dream. After nearly a century of (over)use, the bell curve in intelligence testing continues to impact on children's education and life chances, even if no one can agree what the curve might actually represent.

THE PROBLEM CHILD

'I think I met my first serial killer today,' a friend announced, not long after starting work as a primary-school teacher. 'Every teacher has one!' she insisted, as the rest of the group expressed varying degrees of disbelief. 'That kid you just *know* there's something funny about. And one day, in years to come, you'll turn on the news and see his mugshot staring back at you.' It turned out that little Harry, aged five, had flushed his hamster down the toilet and showed no remorse. Childhood cruelty to animals, my friend pointed out, often appears in the forensic profiles of serial killers. But Harry was five. Was it fair to brand him a problem child at such a young age?

The problem child was a product of the early twentieth century, first in the courts and then in schoolrooms, family homes and on the streets of cities in North America, Europe and Australia. These children were thought to be physically and mentally normal but disruptive, moody or difficult. They might shout, swear, defy their parents, stay out late or shoplift, drink or smoke. Today, we might see this as typical of the normal teenager or pre-teen. In the early twentieth century, though, the 'problem child' aged ten to fifteen was a new worry for parents, psychologists and politicians. These difficult youngsters, it was believed, risked becoming the juvenile delinquents of the future. Just as little Harry was a twenty-first-century serial-killer-in-waiting, in the 1930s twelve-year-old Josie's temper tantrums and fifteen-year-old Malcolm's moodiness were signs of future criminality.[59] Early intervention was key to ensure that the problem child would lead a normal, happy adult life.

Of course, this idea of long-term problems emerging in childhood was not an entirely new one. The child of '"nervous", epileptic, hysterical, hypochondriacal, or unstable' parents should have a heavily regulated upbringing, explained elderly psychiatrist George Fielding Blandford in 1892. By early childhood, the signs of 'nervous inheritance' would appear in night terrors, a fear of the dark, a 'fractious and capricious' temper or a 'violent and passionate' personality.[60] Masturbation, as we've seen, had long been one of the chief dangers to a youth's fragile health. Over-study and competition in education was a new concern, connected to the expansion of the school system. Examination for scholarships, Blandford thought, doomed countless schoolboys to 'all the evil consequences of mental disappointment and sense of failure after years of brain work with all its dangers'.

In 1891, twenty-seven-year-old Frank Wedekind explored the stress schooling caused young people in his first play, *Spring Awakening*. In this coming-of-age tale set in provincial Germany, the teenage Moritz Stiefel fails his exams and commits suicide. His best friend, Melchior Gabor, is sent to a reformatory after raping fourteen-year-old Wendla Bergmann. Bergmann herself dies after a botched abortion. The play was self-published – Wedekind knew full well no theatre would put it on – and wasn't performed in full until 1974.

Spring Awakening differed dramatically from medical depictions of the normal or healthy child in the 1890s because it was written from the perspective of the teenage characters. Adult authority figures are caricatures, with ridiculous names and uncaring attitudes. Parents keep their teenagers in the dark in a misguided effort to preserve their innocence. 'O mother, why didn't you tell me everything?' laments Wendla, astounded to be told that she is pregnant since her mother said she could only have a baby if she was in love.[61] In November 1906, a heavily edited performance finally took place at Berlin's Kammerspiele. The play remained in the theatre's repertoire for two decades and made Wedekind famous. What changed, between 1891 and 1906, that made it possible to talk about teenage angst?

In large part, this was thanks to a new interest in the psychology of childhood.

Perhaps the first person that comes to mind here is Sigmund Freud. Freud's lengthy psychoanalytic case histories delved into his patients' pasts in detail, attributing adult neuroses to childhood experiences, even though Freud himself didn't actually treat children. Certainly, Freud's views on child sexuality were influential in psychoanalytic circles, if vigorously debated by his critics. Popular notions of the abnormal child, however, also converged on the idea that problematic behaviours stemmed from early childhood experiences and should be understood as psychological in origin. This underpinned the child guidance movement of the early twentieth century, first in the US and then in Europe. A bit like baby-weighing clinics, but for older children, the new child guidance centres set up in the 1920s and 1930s provided advice to parents and support for children.

Child guidance emerged from the first juvenile courts, beginning in Illinois in 1899. This created a new understanding of the 'delinquent child'. The delinquent, according to Illinois law, was a child who engaged in a wide range of behaviours: associating with 'vicious or immoral persons', disappearing from home, visiting gambling or drinking establishments or public pool rooms, wandering the streets at night, using 'vile, obscene, vulgar, profane, or indecent language in any public place' or being 'guilty of indecent or lascivious conduct'.[62] While some of these misdemeanours could also result in the arrest of an adult, most would not. Juvenile delinquency laws aimed to regulate a set of behaviours thought to be specifically abnormal in the child. The delinquent was 'more annoying than violent, more socially offensive than criminal'.[63]

Yet the new juvenile delinquent was also thought to be more innocent than Victorian legislators had assumed. He was no longer a born criminal, but a misunderstood and neglected youth, vulnerable to those around him. 'It is as if we ignored a wistful, over-confident creature who walked through our city streets calling out, "I am the spirit of Youth! With me, all things are possible!"' social reformer Jane Addams romanticised. 'We fail to understand what he wants or even to see his doings, although his acts are pregnant with meaning.'[64] Harsh punishment for juvenile crimes was seen as less desirable, since bad behaviour was now thought to reveal hidden mental trauma. The problem child, reformers insisted, needed to be counselled and re-educated rather than punished.

The stories of these children often involved tragedy, especially at the hands of their families. Sophonisba Breckinridge and Edith Abbott's 1912 study of delinquent children in Chicago includes a number of such accounts. Cora's parents drank heavily and kept her out of school to look after her four-year-old brother. The house was full of drunken revellers, and she often roamed the streets late at night to escape. She was brought into court when she was found sleeping 'under the sidewalk'.[65] A thirteen-year-old Polish boy was arrested for stealing grain doors from a railway: his father was ill with pneumonia, and with no food or wood for the fire the boy and his family were starving to death.[66] And when one fifteen-year-old English girl could no longer work in a box factory after her fingers were badly injured, her mother refused to let her stay at home unless she found another way to earn money, forcing her into prostitution.[67]

Breckinridge and Abbott blamed circumstances, and not the children themselves, for their crimes: poverty, misfortune, degeneracy, overcrowding, poor schooling and neighbourhood neglect. All of these weighed most heavily on the poorest families, especially recent immigrants. Like Jane Addams, the pair worried that adults failed to understand children, a view promoted by a new generation of child psychologists. Prominent among these was William Healy, an immigrant child himself when his parents moved to Chicago from England in 1878. Despite dropping out of school to support his family, Healy continued to educate himself and, aged twenty-four, went to Harvard University as a 'special student'. He began to research child psychology but found that the lack of scientific studies of normal physiology and behaviour in children made this challenging.[68]

Healy's textbook on juvenile delinquency, *The Individual Delinquent* (1915), promoted the idea that 'under the shadow of conflict in hidden mental life many a criminalistic tendency is born'.[69] Although late Victorian psychiatrists had assumed only neurotic or unstable children were at risk of delinquency, Healy and his colleagues insisted that *most* children had the potential to become abnormal, if placed in abnormal circumstances. Their circumstances showed 'an effect and a reaction which might well "but for the grace of God", have been duplicated in many a one of us'.[70] This view prompted the growth of the child guidance movement, and 350 clinics were established across the US after the First World War.[71]

This shift in understanding vastly increased the number of people interested in child psychology. In 1918, only three psychologists in the US had a primary research interest in children. By 1937, eighty-one did, while in 1956, 'nearly a thousand members and fellows of the APA [American Psychological Association] indicate the child, or work with children, as their first interest'.[72] The same thing happened in England and Australia, as the view that abnormal behaviour emerged from childhood experiences became widespread.[73]

By reinterpreting the delinquent child, early twentieth-century American reformers re-shaped the idea of the

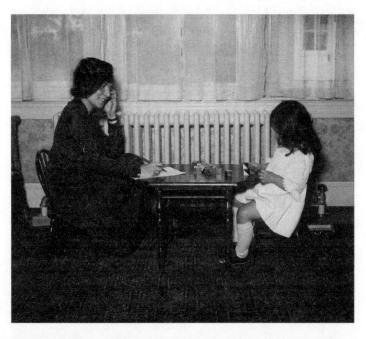

A child with an unidentified psychologist or social worker at Washington Child Guidance Clinic, 1931.

normal child. The Victorians had assumed that only certain children – like James Henry Pullen – were mentally abnormal, an accident of birth. Early twentieth-century psychologists assumed that *many* children, although born 'normal', were at risk of psychological maladjustment due to their circumstances. After the Second World War this view of child psychology changed further. *All* children, post-war psychologists suggested, were potentially abnormal. And their parents' actions, it seemed, posed the biggest threat to a child's emotional and psychological health.

THE RISE OF EMOTIONAL HEALTH

'This is Laura in her garden at home.' So began one of the most influential films of post-war childhood development. Two-and-a-half-year-old Laura was a bright and active girl, with loving parents thrilled by her rapid development. 'They say with a certain pride,' the viewer is told, '"It takes a lot to make Laura cry."' The film – *A Two-Year-Old Goes to Hospital* – was made by social worker James Robertson and psychologist John Bowlby in 1952. It was a detailed documentary of Laura's eight-day stay in hospital for treatment of umbilical hernia, a 'commonplace' occurrence, as Bowlby put it. It was 'simply the story of a child of 2½ years who spends eight days in hospital for a minor operation and who frets a good deal of this time'.[74]

By laying stress on the significance of Laura's fretting, *A Two-Year-Old Goes to Hospital* claimed that even normal distress in childhood might lead to emotional disturbance. For perhaps the first time, the child's emotional responses took centre stage. The film has no sound – we hear Laura's words only through the narrator, while watching the child's tears. We are not usually told what nurses or doctors do or say to soothe her, making their efforts appear distant and alien. The film's impact is increased by the fact that we are constantly told that Laura is an unusual child. Although she was apparently selected randomly by a hospital clerk, the narrator calls her 'quite unusual in being able to control the expression of her feelings'.[75] This emphasises how greatly affected Laura is, encouraging us to look beyond what is immediately visible.

It may seem obvious to us now, seventy years later, that Laura would be upset by being left in hospital by her parents. For a 1950s audience, however, the film was eye-opening. Presented from the perspective of a child, it turned adult assumptions on their head. At the time, parental visiting in hospitals was often limited because it caused sudden distress in children who had seemed calm. Robertson and Bowlby contradicted this wisdom, claiming that it was not, after all, a good sign when Laura did not cry or demand attention. It was not evidence that she was coping with separation but of withdrawal: her 'fretting' or 'protest' behaviour had shifted into 'despair'.[76]

This despair, a second stage of separation, was more dangerous than the first. A boy called Roddy was parted from his mother for three years between the ages of one and four while in hospital and a tuberculosis sanatorium, and withdrew from all interpersonal relationships.[77] His relationship with his mother remained difficult for 'at least' two and a half years after his return home.[78] Laura, Roddy and other children separated from their mothers were not unstable or difficult children. Their emotional responses were to be expected – they 'gradually became affected as a normal child must'. Yet these changes were nonetheless interpreted as dangerous, causing the child to become emotionally unstable. Bowlby compared infant separations to older troubled children like Desmond, aged eleven, whose violent outbursts included trying to set his therapist's chair on fire, burn her hair and stockings, and strangle her. The fretting of a toddler, Bowlby concluded, showed 'the beginning of that disruption of the capacity to make love relations which we saw in Desmond', a bold conclusion that terrified generations of parents.[79]

In the US, Harry Harlow's famous primate experiments reinforced Bowlby's theory. Orphaned baby monkeys were given two mother surrogates: a wire frame mother, and one padded with soft cloth. Half the infants were bottle-fed from the wire mother, and half from the cloth mother. Regardless of where their food came from, all the baby monkeys spent most of their time clinging to the cloth mother. Harlow's experiments became world-famous. They were perfect for the new post-war television audience. Documentary clips show huge-eyed baby monkeys cuddling their mother surrogate, and even nuzzling and 'kissing' her face. When Harlow described this as 'love', it was easy for an audience to anthropomorphise what they saw. The wire mother was 'biologically adequate but psychologically inept', according to Harlow, making the cloth mother – with her exaggerated smile and big eyes – a visual representation of maternal monkey love.

Harlow's experiments provided ideal ammunition for Bowlby's attachment theory, as it became known in 1956.[80]

They seemed to prove that baby monkeys – and, by Harlow's extension, humans – needed physical contact with a soft mother surrogate to develop emotionally. When isolated wire-reared monkeys were placed in a playroom with others of the same age, the researchers 'were just completely blown away in terms of their total lack of emotional regulation and any sort of normal social repertoires'.[81] Yet while Bowlby had assumed that the mother played the major role in a child's developing emotions – 'when Laura is tired or hurt, it's her mother she turns to for comfort' – Harlow disagreed. His mother surrogates did nothing but warm and comfort the baby monkey – they were successful even when they did not feed it. 'It is cheering', Harlow concluded, 'to realize that the American male is physically endowed with all the really essential equipment to compete with the American female on equal terms in one essential activity: the rearing of infants.'[82] If a cloth surrogate could provide comfort and security, then all human parents were equal.

Not that anyone else seemed to notice this potential. Mothers were still widely blamed for going to work, as they had been by health visitors on the lookout for verminous children in the 1920s. Now, however, it was the emotional needs of their infants these 'wire mothers' were neglecting and not their physical health. As the American childcare guru Dr Spock put it, a mother 'deciding' to go to work had quite simply failed to recognise the needs of her infant.[83] In Britain, Ronald Illingworth thought that a mother generally resorted to a nanny 'because she cannot be bothered to bring [… a child] up herself or because she thinks it is fashionable', ignoring the fact that mothers might need or want to work and require support from others to care for a child.[84] The assumption remained that the normal development of the child was the mother's lone responsibility.

FROM SHYNESS TO HYPERACTIVITY

'All normal children have behaviour problems,' Illingworth stressed. 'It is wrong to think that children with these problems are in any way abnormal, naughty, nervous or maladjusted.' It was usually the parents who needed to change and not the child, who needed – as Bowlby had said – constant love and security, especially 'when he is least lovable'.[85] Among the now normal behaviour problems of children in the post-war years – refusing to eat or sleep, bed-wetting, temper tantrums, thumb-sucking, masturbation, anxiety, shyness and stuttering – one thing was newly of interest: hyperactivity.

ADHD – or attention deficit hyperactivity disorder – remains controversial today, in part because it is such a recent addition to defining the normal child. Before 1957, hyperactivity was not generally seen as clinically important. It was the withdrawn and quiet child who was the object of child guidance: Bowlby's Laura, suffering from maternal deprivation. After 1957, however, concern began to shift from the shy, neurotic child to the 'excessively active' one.[86] From the start, hyperactivity was associated with 'normal' children. As psychiatrists Maurice Laufer and Eric Denhoff put it in 1957, 'hyperkinetic behaviour syndrome' was not something associated only with a few but was 'a common behaviour disorder' among children of 'normal intelligence'.[87] By 1962, it was thought to be one of the most widespread behaviour problems in children in the US, and in 1968, after it was added to DSM-II, it was thought to exist in epidemic proportions.[88] The acronym ADHD appeared only in 1987 (preceded by ADD – attention deficit disorder – in 1980).

The extremely rapid rise of this new diagnosis was driven by a range of factors: the growth of the pharmaceutical industry and direct-to-consumer advertising, the rise of parent lobbying groups, a new approach to psychiatry that focused on symptom management, and, later, fear about the use of additives in children's diets. According to historian Matthew Smith, the Cold War formed the perfect environment for ADHD to flourish. The post-Sputnik panic sparked calls to improve the US education system. Child-centred learning would be replaced by a more rigid system, to ensure American science could rival Soviet Russia. Children were expected to stay in school longer and to learn more while they were there. Disruptive children were increasingly targeted. They were considered harmful not only to their own learning but to their classmates; meanwhile the newly introduced school counsellor would help to identify and treat these 'hyperactive' children.[89]

From the beginning, diagnosis of hyperactivity was based on class and race. In the 1960s, poor and ethnic-minority children in the US were more likely to be diagnosed with the stigmatising 'mild mental retardation' while their wealthier, white counterparts were described as hyperkinetic or with 'minimal brain dysfunction' – even when children displayed exactly the same symptoms.[90] While the language used was less starkly offensive than the Victorians'

racial hierarchies of development, the system remained
deeply racist. In Britain, Grenadian writer Bernard Coard
was horrified by the over-representation of Black children
in ESN ('educationally subnormal') schools. When West
Indian children struggled with emotional or environmen-
tal challenges, such as experiencing racism, their behaviour
and difficulties in learning were classed by their white
teachers not as normal responses to external problems but
as mental retardation.[91]

In contrast, by the late twentieth century, ADHD was
inextricably attached to the white middle class, the very
group deemed to epitomise the 'normal', making diagnosis
almost a status symbol. A 1997 cartoon of a white baby with
a silver spoon in its mouth mockingly asked parents: 'What
does your healthy, normal, perfect, little darling need to get
ahead in life? A small disability to qualify for special aid!'[92]

Diagnosis of hyperactivity in children took off dramatically in post-war America. A simple, neurological
explanation with an even more simple solution in the prescription of Ritalin proved enduringly popular to parents,
teachers and psychiatrists, despite the significant side effects
of this medication. It was easier, after all, to turn to drugs
than the post-war social psychology promoted by Bowlby
and Illingworth. By 1993, more than 3 million American
children were on Ritalin and ADHD was beginning to be
diagnosed in adulthood. The diagnosis was also spreading
around the world, much to the concern of some of its early
advocates. Psychologist Keith Conners, who developed the
first standard rating scales for hyperactivity in the 1960s,
asked the *British Medical Journal* to include a warning in
his own obituary about the overdiagnosis of the disorder,

calling it a 'national disaster of dangerous proportions'.[93]

We are all used to searching for explanations for behaviour, and sometimes a psychiatric diagnosis offers an attractive one, especially when we *know* that our child isn't bad or lazy and need a way to prove it to others. Medication may be helpful, just as therapy can be. When we look at the historical shift, however, from exploring a child's environment and relationships to a reliance on medication, we can see another side to these changes. The lesson from the Bowlby era was supposed to be that all normal children can easily experience behavioural problems. The twenty-first-century view suggests that, with pharmaceutical assistance, difficult children can just as quickly be 'fixed'. But does that really get to the root of the problem? When we label the behaviour of children as hyperactive, autistic or otherwise different, it becomes all too easy to ignore the social factors that shape that child's experiences – and continue to do so, whatever medication or treatment they might go on to take. It's much easier, after all, to dose a child up on Ritalin than to change a school system to suit different styles of learning. It's easier to label a Black child as educationally subnormal than to recognise – and deal with – the racism woven into our institutional structures. Of course, struggling parents and distressed children may well need medical or psychological support. But that shouldn't blind us to this important context.

NORMAL CHILDREN OR ABNORMAL PARENTS?

In his mid-thirties, Tyler Page decided to explore his life with ADHD in a graphic novel. Looking at his childhood medical records decades after he was first diagnosed aged nine in 1985, Page found they raised more questions than they answered. The simplistic life story he remembered – a straightforward medical tale of diagnosis, medication and improvement – was not quite so simple after all. 'I was reminded of things I'd forgotten,' he wrote, 'chiefly, the connection between the knife incident [slashing up a school bus seat] and uncovering our deeper family problems. In my memory, they were separate incidents.' His environment and childhood experiences, Page decided, were not unimportant in understanding his symptoms. He concluded, however, that ADHD was a useful diagnosis because it helped him understand and manage his experiences. But that didn't mean it didn't continue to raise questions. 'Did being on meds affect who I've become?' he wondered. 'And most importantly, what does it mean for my children?'[94]

Having children might cause us to re-evaluate our own lives as well as theirs. Not so long ago, a close friend told me he was thinking about getting tested for autism. Although he had long worried about certain traits in his own behaviour, it was his relationship with his young daughter that had sparked new concerns. Your mum and dad might indeed fuck you up, but they have probably also spent half their lives worrying about it. For the Victorians, the main way that parents could damage their children was through their biology – a neurotic or damaged inheritance, often framed in terms of race or class. In the Edwardian era, a child's environment became more important. This did not, however, mean that parents were off the hook – especially working-class mothers, blamed for the abnormally small size of their infants or 'verminous' offspring.

From this emerged the problem child of the early twentieth century. Again, 'problem parents' were often blamed for these 'abnormal children': neglect, poor care or simple poverty might cause childhood troubles, social workers assumed. Yet, as the child guidance movement grew and childhood psychology took centre stage, even the 'well-cared-for' child became at risk of instability. And sometimes there was little parents could do to turn the tide. Would Laura's parents have been able to prevent her operation or persuade the hospital to change its policies to stop the upset of separation? It's unlikely. Yet they and countless other parents began to worry about the emotional health of their children, seeking out and identifying behaviour problems because problems were what they now expected to see.

When I spoke to my friend about his fears, I thought back to a little girl I met while working on a farm as a teenager, the first time I had ever heard of the diagnosis of autism. Even at the time, I marvelled about the lack of difference between us, other than a few years in age. She was kind to me in a difficult period of my life, and her words always stayed with me. Would I have thought differently of her if I had known more about the label she had been given? I remember too a primary school visit to a museum I once worked at, how impressed we all were with the way the class engaged in complex issues and came up with creative ideas. Afterwards, the teacher told us that these were the naughtier and less able children: the others had been sent on a more popular trip. She too was surprised by the way they had responded when no one knew that they were not thought the most gifted children in the school. Labels are an easy thing to obtain but far harder to shake off. They might help us to explain and understand, but they can also limit us. Would I have bothered with the years it took me to learn to hug people or look them in the eye if I had thought it was hardwired into my DNA to be incapable of doing so?

What is average or common in childhood varies immensely. When we use one group to interpret others – taking a white, middle-class lifestyle as 'normal', as in the Army Alpha IQ test – those from other backgrounds will certainly be shown to differ. This has often, as we have seen, led to those who don't meet these arbitrary criteria being judged abnormal. But what if it's the environment that needs to change? Social interventions such as free school meals and vitamins, for example, made some previously visible 'abnormalities' simply disappear. Educational support, Alfred Binet thought, would improve the IQ of less able children. Perhaps, then, some of our kids' behaviours and abilities *are* linked to genes and biology. But, certainly, very many of them are not.

7

IS SOCIETY NORMAL?

On 29 January 2020, I went into work with a cough. I'd been ill since soon after New Year and, although my cold was coming to an end, a frustrating cough persisted. Just before lunchtime I sat down with a colleague, but a coughing fit interrupted the start of our meeting. Her eyes narrowed.

'You haven't got coronavirus, have you?' she asked.

We both laughed. At the time, the idea seemed unimaginable. That week was the first time I'd thought seriously about the spread of the new outbreak, even if it never crossed my mind that I might have it.

Five weeks later, on Wednesday 11 March, the World Health Organization announced a coronavirus pandemic. By this time Covid-19 (as it had become widely known) had reached 114 countries and killed more than 4,000 people. In Britain, many of us knew the declaration of a pandemic was coming: if anything, it seemed rather late. But no one appeared unduly concerned. 'You just need to make sure you wash your hands,' colleagues and neighbours alike said dismissively. 'It's common sense!'

The weekend after the pandemic was announced I was due to visit my sister and her two-week-old baby, my second niece. She texted a few days before my visit asking if I could come a bit sooner. It was, after all, the week everything was changing. Workplaces across Europe began to send staff home. Italy – now the epicentre of a European outbreak – was in total lockdown and other countries began to shut their borders. Tourism ended. Several friends were forced to cancel eagerly awaited trips abroad. One went to Chile anyway and almost didn't return.

People with any symptoms were urged to self-isolate. So were those considered vulnerable – over-seventies, people with long-term health conditions, pregnant women. My parents, arriving at my sister's house for a brief reunion the day I left for London, returned to their tiny Dorset hamlet to prepare for seclusion. My mum cheerfully told me that she planned to take apart the jigsaw I had given her for Christmas and begin it all over again. No one anticipated how long lockdown would, in fact, last.

When I travelled back through London the weekend after the pandemic was declared, Oxford Street was still full of shoppers. Face masks remained a rarity. Underneath, however, things were starting to unravel. Supermarkets around the world sold out of toilet roll, pasta and tinned tomatoes. My Tesco delivery – booked weeks earlier – was cancelled a few hours before it was due to arrive. The next available slot was a fortnight later. I was lucky to get one at all.

Bigger cracks were beginning to show across society. The National Health Service, already over-stretched, struggled to deal with an influx of patients. In care homes things were even worse, as hospital patients were discharged without testing. Staff made their own masks, put rotas in place for dealing with infected patients, and were forced to quarantine with the mildest of symptoms in the absence of testing. The lowest paid, on insecure contracts, couldn't afford to quarantine at all. By 28 March 2020 there had been 759 deaths in British hospitals from Covid-19.[1] As this book goes to press, over two years later, 175,000 people have died in the UK alone.

Pubs, restaurants, gyms and shops closed. People lost their jobs or were placed on furlough, a government scheme paying 80 per cent of the usual wage. Even for those who received it – by no means everyone – it wasn't always enough to get by, and use of food banks soared. Some people struggled to pay the rent and worried about losing their homes. The closure of schools revealed a digital divide across the nation. Not all children could take part in online learning; some had no home broadband or computer. The government promised a million laptops to disadvantaged children, and promptly forgot about them.

Society changed beyond all recognition. It shouldn't have seemed normal. But, in an odd sort of way, it did. 'Ordinary is what you are used to,' Aunt Lydia says in Margaret Atwood's dystopian novel *The Handmaid's Tale*. 'This may not seem ordinary to you now, but after a time it will. It will become ordinary.'[2] After months of regulations, changes to the restrictions we live under were met with a weary sigh. We began to get used to this new normal. It became ordinary.

That's not to say that the problems and inequalities revealed by the Covid-19 pandemic no longer shock us.

The pandemic has exposed many flaws that already existed within our society. It has shown us just how fragile the threads that bind us together are, and how easily everything can be turned on its head. The things many people assumed to be the natural order are no longer so certain. The nine-to-five office day. Job security. Universal education. Consumerism. Healthcare. Individual freedom. Once upon a time all these things seemed quite normal. Then, one day, these certainties were suddenly and unexpectedly snatched away.

But perhaps, after all, what this really suggests is that none of those things were ever quite as straightforward or as normal as we were led to believe. The structures of our society – our laws, our customs, and our expectations – are just as historically constructed as our ideas about a normal body or mind.

THE (COLONIAL) ORIGINS OF THE SOCIAL ORGANISM

The Sign of Four (1890), the second Sherlock Holmes mystery by Arthur Conan Doyle, introduced Holmes's infamous cocaine habit, as well as Dr Watson's future wife, Mary Morstan. It also drew on the science of the normal. 'Let me recommend this book – one of the most remarkable ever penned,' Holmes inexplicably tells Watson, just as he is about to dash out to investigate something. 'It is Winwood Reade's *Martyrdom of Man*.'[3] Although Watson was too distracted by thoughts of his future wife to read it,* Holmes returned to Reade's popular yet controversial evolutionary history of civilisation towards the close of the mystery, attributing to him the idea that 'while the individual man is an insoluble puzzle, in the aggregate he becomes a mathematical certainty'.[4] Of course, this notion had been circulating in statistical circles ever since Quetelet. Reade's 1872 book, already in its seventeenth edition by 1890, brought the idea to a much wider audience. It also cemented the belief that society itself *was* this aggregate.

The 'social organism', as grumpy philosopher Herbert Spencer called it, was a new entity that emerged from the science of the normal.[5] Society became cast as a living creature, the cells in its body made up of the individuals living and working within it.[6] This implied that society, like each human being, was a natural entity. Charles Darwin proposed that the evolution of society was a natural process in his *The Descent of Man* (1871), drawing on the work of anthropologists who equated non-Western peoples with 'primitive man'.[7] These 'armchair anthropologists' – so called because they used the data other travellers had gathered, sitting in their plush living rooms to write up the results – assumed that the social customs and habits of small tribes were the same as those of past societies uncovered in archaeological excavations.

This belief supported the pre-existing notion that non-Western societies were less evolved than white Western

* When I tried to follow Holmes's recommendation in my early twenties, like Watson I struggled to focus on *The Martyrdom of Man*. Unlike Watson, I wondered what on earth the book had to do with the case at hand or, indeed, any of Holmes's detective work. Presumably it had recently made a big impact on Conan Doyle himself.

ones. 'A general survey of the lower races', the well-respected anthropologist Edward Burnett Tylor generalised, 'shows that their selfish and malevolent tendencies are stronger in proportion to their unselfish and benevolent tendencies, than in higher grades of culture.'[8] Darwin used a similar link to propose that the development of social instincts in history had led to the dominance of co-operative groups over selfish ones.[9] Then, through a curiously vague mixture of inherited habits, sexual selection and social censure, the individuals with the most social feeling made their way to the top of the social order.

As we have seen time and again, this assumption by white Western scientists – that the society they lived in was the best one – used the concept of the normal as a means of establishing cultural and material dominance. 'Our government has been of late engaged in putting down the criminal clans or castes of British India,' Tylor remarked; 'clans whose moral law naturally seems to themselves virtuous, but which the authorities deem incompatible with the well-being of society.'[10] Normal was not, here, what seemed 'natural' to a particular group of people, but externally imposed by a dominant culture. Tylor was referring to the Criminal Tribes Act of 1871, a repressive law which demanded the registration and control of certain groups across India, due to the belief that they were habitually criminal.

The entire population of so-called British India was required by law to monitor these groups, especially in isolated villages where the British authorities rarely ventured. Thirteen million people were affected by this law until its repeal in 1947 when India finally gained independence.[11]

One such 'tribe' was the *hijra* or *hijda*, a group of gender-non-conforming people, today formally recognised on the Indian subcontinent as a third gender. It seems that this group had been granted an official right to beg in the eighteenth century, and a legitimate claim on public revenue. According to historian Laurence Preston, it was these rights that the British objected to and which led to the *hijra* being classified as a criminal tribe.[12] While the identification of the group as abnormal ostensibly occurred for economic reasons, it was their practices that were cast as an affront to society. A 'man' becoming a 'Hijera and appearing in public in the garb of a woman', wrote the Commissioner of Satara in 1855, was 'such a breach of morality and of the rules of public decency as to justify the present Government

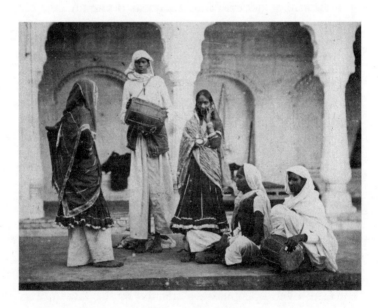

Photograph of a group of *hijra* with musical instruments, India, c.1860s.

in at once withholding their continuance'.[13]

While the *hijra* were already classed as a problem by the British government in India, other groups became so in the aftermath of the Indian rebellion of 1857. Indeed, the solution to the Holmes mystery *The Sign of Four* emerged from this context of colonial repression. It turns out that an Englishman named Jonathan Small acquired treasure in the aftermath of the 'great mutiny', when, as he describes in starkly racist terms, 'two hundred thousand black devils let loose, and the country was a perfect hell'.[14] As in other British reports from the time, Conan Doyle represented the rebellion as an unleashing of primitive tendencies, which infects Small too when he joins forces with two Sikhs to murder a wealthy Indian merchant and steal his treasure.

Ultimately, however, Small is not to blame for the death in London, thirty years after the events in India, of another Englishman. This murder was perpetrated by Small's friend Tonga, an Andaman Islander, a 'little bloodthirsty imp' who 'thought he had done something very clever in killing him'.[15] Once again, non-Western people are presented – in fiction as in science – as dangerous to Western civilisation. And the fictional Tonga's lack of remorse – despite his loyalty to Small – reflects Tylor's claim that 'savage laws' were framed around small groups, 'restraining murder and theft within the tribe, but permitting them outside'.[16] By this logic, small tribes, village-led communities and nomadic peoples were deemed by their colonisers to be dangerous to wider society, and hence often cruelly repressed.

These sweeping generalisations were, of course, created by well-educated and well-off men from white, Western, industrialised societies – as were the laws devised and implemented to enforce them. They entered popular fiction, indicating how widespread racist and colonialist assumptions about social norms and customs were. It was not until the twentieth century that anthropologists began to view different social structures, and the legal frameworks supporting them, as culturally relative. For Victorian scientists, a particular society, like an individual, could be healthy or unhealthy, normal or abnormal, desirable or undesirable. Societies evolved, they thought, just as individuals did, and the most normal of societies was that in which they found themselves. What they saw elsewhere was often what they expected, supporting a preconceived hierarchy of civilisation, while their customs and practices became the yardstick by which they judged the rest of the world.

THE MIDDLE FILLING OF THE COMMUNITY PIE

Despite – or perhaps because of – this, normal Western society itself went largely unexamined until January 1924, when Robert and Helen Lynd arrived in Muncie, Indiana, with a small team of research assistants. The young couple had recently married and Middletown – as their study became known – was their first joint social science project. The Lynds stayed in Muncie until June 1925, studying the lives of the townspeople through observation and countless surveys. Their description focused on what was usual in that society. The very term 'middle' implied that the usual was also some kind of average, even when such things couldn't be measured statistically (what, after all, is the average job or the average lifestyle?). When *Middletown* was eventually published in 1929 it became a surprise bestseller, going through six printings in the first year of publication, astounding sales figures for a social science study.[17]

What was it that fascinated the American public about Middletown? For one thing, the study was about so-called 'normal' people. Just as psychologists were moving towards studying the everyday in the decades after the First World War, the Lynds' study was one of the first anthropological investigations of Western social life. Of course, Émile Durkheim, the grandfather of sociology, had also set great store in identifying what was normal. The 'principal object of all sciences of life, whether individual or social,' he claimed in 1895, 'is to define and explain the normal state and to distinguish it from its opposite'.[18] To decide if an

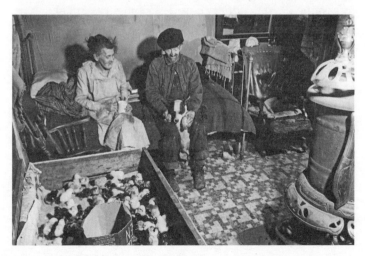

Scott and Lizabelle Brandenburg sitting on a bed in their one-room shack in Muncie, Indiana (Margaret Bourke-White for *Life* magazine, 1937).

attribute or custom was normal in society, the sociologist first had to determine that it occurred frequently. They then had to look at the conditions that had brought the custom into being, and see if these still applied: in other words, did the custom have some social function or use? If both things were satisfied then the 'social fact' – as Durkheim called it – was normal. The normal became, at one and the same time, the thing that happened to exist most frequently *and* what ought to exist in society. This leap from description to judgement is one that happens time and again where normal society is concerned.

It is not surprising, then, that although the Lynds saw normal society as relative, this was not at all how Middletown became understood. The Lynds wanted to examine 1920s American life as 'simply the form which human behaviour under this particular set of conditions has come to assume'.[19] Yet, rather than describing a particular type of society, or showing that norms were relative, the book – and the town on which it was based – quickly came to stand 'as shorthand for contemporary America and a summation of "who we are"'.[20] While the Lynds had been clear that their study could 'only with caution be applied to other cities or to American life in general', readers and reviewers leapt on the idea of Middletown as a mirror, reflecting ordinary America.[21] During the 1930s, Middletown so summed up typical America that advertisers flocked to Muncie, viewing it as the ideal testing ground for products intended to appeal to 'Mr and Mrs John Citizen of Middletown, USA'.[22]

However, as historian Sarah Igo points out in her study of the 'averaged American', Muncie was not actually all that typical. Ninety per cent of cities of a similar size had a greater proportion of women in paid employment.[23] Muncie was also abnormal in its lack of ethnic diversity. In Muncie, 92 per cent of the population were of 'native American stock', said the Lynds, by which they meant white people born in the US. This figure was higher than in almost any other city in the Midwest.[24] Compounding this difference, the Lynds made the decision to investigate *only* the white population of Muncie. No answers from the city's 2,000 or so African Americans (5.6 per cent of the population) were included in Middletown's tables.[25] As in the case of Norma, typical woman, the white American was used to set a standard, generating a skewed set of expectations that would later come to be imposed on those – Black and foreign-born residents – whose data had not been included in defining norms in the first place.

This deliberate avoidance of race also altered the way in which the lives of the white population of Muncie were understood. The Lynds admitted that some 3,500 citizens (a full 10 per cent of the population) were members of the Ku Klux Klan, and that the Klan 'controlled Muncie's city government and led boycotts against Catholic and Jewish businesses'.[26] These comments, however, came late in the book, kept quite separate from the discussions of work, family and home life. The Lynds did not consider how the lives of all citizens were shaped by lines of segregation or that white American cultural norms were created by the systematic exclusion of other groups.[27] Instead they exacerbated this exclusionary practice by removing Muncie's Black population from their study. Just as the Victorians had held a particular type of white, Western society as 'normal' amid the diverse cultures of the world, Middletown cemented the view that a particular group of people were representative of industrialised America.

Although the Lynds ignored race as a factor shaping American society, they did write a lot about the impact of class on Muncie's residents. Whether or not someone was born into the business class or the working class, they asserted, was 'the most significant single cultural factor tending to influence what one does all day long throughout one's life; whom one marries; when one gets up in the morning; whether one belongs to the Holy Roller or Presbyterian church; or drives a Ford or a Buick'.[28] Changes in working life had exacerbated class divisions in Muncie over the last few decades. Mechanisation in factories and foundries, for example, was wiping out job satisfaction for the working class, as well as making life harder for older workers.[29] Increasing numbers of working-class women worked because they had to, despite being paid significantly less than men.[30]

But while the Lynds saw class division everywhere, the popular notion of middle-of-the-road Middletown implied to many readers that it was the *middle* class who were representative of the community. When *Life* magazine sent a photographer, Margaret Bourke-White, to capture Muncie in 1937, local people were outraged by her pictures of the homes of poorer residents. 'They didn't show the average Muncie family – only extremes,' a local journalist complained. 'She "shot" the upper crust and the lower (soaked) crust but left out the middle-filling,' objected another resident, asserting that the middle was 'the most important part of any community-pie'.[31]

This idea that the middle class was especially 'normal' was not entirely new. The growth of the bourgeoisie in the late Victorian era had already shaped the 'average man' as the middle-class professional. After Middletown, however, this view of middle-class normality became widespread. Normal American society, post-Middletown, was widely assumed to be represented by the white, native-born, town-dwelling middle-class resident. It didn't matter that the bulk of the population didn't fit this description – a full 70 per cent of Muncie residents had been categorised as working class by the Lynds, after all. The middle filling of the community pie might not be particularly thick, but this middling sort nonetheless became the American norm. We still hear the terms 'Middle America' or 'Middle England' today, perhaps with more disparaging undertones, to refer to a particular group of people: white, middle class and politically conservative. These have never been the most common type of people in any society, yet their role as guardians of the 'normal' has continually reinforced their cultural dominance, along with the conservative values that they are thought to represent. And, of course, this only serves to further marginalise those who, for whatever reason, do not fit this norm.

LEADERS OF THE FUTURE

In September 1936, John F. Kennedy enrolled at Harvard University. Born into a wealthy and politically connected family, the young Kennedy was an obvious candidate for a study that began two years after he arrived: the Harvard

Grant Study.[32] This scientific project aimed to measure every characteristic of so-called 'normal young men': their bodies, minds, health, personalities, backgrounds and achievements.[33] Participants were most definitely not average men.* In the first place, they all attended an elite university. And from that unique pool of people were selected those students deemed most psychologically and physically well and who had reached a certain level of academic attainment. Two-thirds had been to private schools, and a full third came from families with an income of more than $15,000 a year (the median annual income for a man in the US in 1940 was $956). They were probably – since the study didn't specify – all white. Even with this rigorous pre-selection, the Harvard 'normal' men showed significant variation on almost every physical and mental characteristic, from body temperature to personality. 'The only thing that made them "normal"', notes historian Anna Creadick, 'was their a priori selection into a category with that label.'[34]

The claim that these young men were normal was based on a range of assumptions about the category itself. Normal, according to the Harvard Grant Study, was neither the statistical average nor someone in perfect health. It meant 'the *balanced* person whose combination of traits of all sorts allows him to function effectively in a variety of ways'.[35] This normal standard was based exclusively on a particular group, even more limited than that represented by Middletown: white, upper middle or upper class, able-bodied,

* The Grant Study continues to this day, running alongside the Glueck Study, which is made up of 456 men who grew up in inner-city Boston. The publications examined here, however, all focus on the Grant Study, as an investigation into 'normal young men'.

neurotypical and particularly 'masculine' men.[36] These young men, the study claimed, would be the leaders of the future: an assertion made on no other basis than the belief that they were, well, 'normal'.

Of course, in Kennedy's case at least, the study did correctly identify a leader. Twenty-one years after graduating from Harvard, in 1961, John F. Kennedy became the thirty-fifth president of the United States. But how much of this selection was a self-fulfilling prophecy? 'Leaders of the people should rise from among those who are well and fit,' the Harvard report concluded, using the language of eugenics to associate normalcy with social and political power.[37] A popular book based on the study, written by physical anthropologist Earnest Hooton, went still further, recommending 'measures taken to prevent obvious genetic inferiors from having off-spring'.[38] Not only was the normal created by emphasising certain characteristics and excluding others, it was used to justify an ongoing process of discrimination, even as the Second World War drew to a close.

Kennedy's assassination, after just under three years as president of the US, left something of a rose-tinted legacy. A Democrat who supported the civil rights movement, he nonetheless personified a certain 'normal' America, in which leaders were identified by a set of traits, which made them appear particularly 'well and fit'. In Kennedy's era, the voices of those who had been excluded from the boundaries of 'normal society' also became increasingly loud – the world saw the growth of, among other things, the Black civil rights movement, gay rights, anti-psychiatry and a new social model of disability. But the slow pace of change in many parts of public life suggests that it is not enough for the comfortable to recognise the exclusion of others. Instead, across Western society and beyond, we all need to recognise that the normal ideal itself is not a natural entity, but something that has been socially and politically engineered over the past centuries.

Let's go back to the 'WEIRD'ness of Western societies, where we began. Indeed, the WEIRD undergraduates described by Joseph Henrich, Steven Heine and Ara Norenzayan in 2010 are a very similar group to the young men making up the 1930s Harvard Grant Study. Their results in psychological (and medical and sociological) tests have somehow become viewed as 'representative' of human beings in general, even though their lives and experiences are in a minority. If enough of us learn to privilege those experiences as a normal standard, then we are likely to judge our own lives by them whether we meet the criteria or not. As happens when we measure our bodies and minds against a fictitious average, we are set an impossible goal to follow. In the case of society, the average often isn't even something created by the statistics of our fellow citizens; instead, it's an ideal that serves a range of political and cultural purposes.

'The Western conception of the person as a bounded, unique, more or less integrated motivational and cognitive universe', pointed out renowned anthropologist Clifford Geertz in 1974, is 'a rather peculiar idea within the context of the world's cultures.'[39] In other words, thinking of yourself in individualistic terms, as distinctly separate from other individuals – a common belief in Western capitalist societies – is not all that normal. I remember finding this idea very hard to grasp during my psychology A level. It seemed so obvious to me that I was a separate, independent unit from others. Yet, when we think about it, most situations in our lives can be interpreted relationally. In some languages, like Vietnamese or Japanese, pronouns change depending on the relationship with the person being addressed. The self may not be a fixed entity but differs depending on who one is with.*

Anyway, even Westerners may be less individual than we think we are. Certainly, a host of psychology studies in the post-war era cast doubt on this matter. By far the most famous was Stanley Milgram's study of obedience, inspired by the young psychologist's graduate work on conformity with Solomon Asch. Asch found that people could be influenced to give incorrect answers to simple questions when they were part of a group that consistently gave the wrong answers. Milgram's study was rather more headline-grabbing, using a realistic-looking but completely harmless electric shock machine. His experiment employed actors in the role of experimenter and learner. The experimenter told the real subject that they were acting as the teacher in a study on learning and punishment, and had them read out a series of memory tests. For every incorrect answer the learner gave, the teacher was to give him an electric shock

---

* The way things are expressed in different languages is fascinating. In Russian, for example, one doesn't say 'I have a friend' but 'by me exists a friend', which seems to make more literal sense when you think about it. The friend is the subject of the Russian sentence, whereas 'I' is the subject of the English sentence. This says a lot about the 'individualism complex' of WEIRD people, as Henrich puts it. Russia is kind of middling in the individualism scale on most of Henrich's maps; North America, Europe and Australia tend towards the most individualistic. Joseph Henrich, *The Weirdest People in the World* (New York and London: Allen Lane, 2020), 26–7.

Public Announcement

WE WILL PAY YOU $4.00 FOR
ONE HOUR OF YOUR TIME

Persons Needed for a Study of Memory

*We will pay five hundred New Haven men to help us complete a scientific study of memory and learning. The study is being done at Yale University.
*Each person who participates will be paid $4.00 (plus 50c carfare) for approximately 1 hour's time. We need you for only one hour: there are no further obligations. You may choose the time you would like to come (evenings, weekdays, or weekends).

*No special training, education, or experience is needed. We want:

Factory workers	Businessmen	Construction workers
City employees	Clerks	Salespeople
Laborers	Professional people	White-collar workers
Barbers	Telephone workers	Others

All persons must be between the ages of 20 and 50. High school and college students cannot be used.
*If you meet these qualifications, fill out the coupon below and mail it now to Professor Stanley Milgram, Department of Psychology, Yale University, New Haven. You will be notified later of the specific time and place of the study. We reserve the right to decline any application.
*You will be paid $4.00 (plus 50c carfare) as soon as you arrive at the laboratory.

TO:
PROF. STANLEY MILGRAM, DEPARTMENT OF PSYCHOLOGY, YALE UNIVERSITY, NEW HAVEN, CONN. I want to take part in this study of memory and learning. I am between the ages of 20 and 50. I will be paid $4.00 (plus 50c carfare) if I participate.

NAME (Please Print)...................................

ADDRESS ....

TELEPHONE NO. .... Best time to call you ....

AGE........OCCUPATION..................... SEX......
CAN YOU COME:

WEEKDAYS .... EVENINGS ......WEEKENDS.........

Original 1963 advertisement for Milgram's experiment, asking for volunteers for a 'memory study'. These volunteers were actually subjects in his experiment on obedience to authority.

– gradually increasing to the maximum possible, 450 volts. Marked 'XXX' on the machine, this was two levels above the already ominous 'Danger: Severe Shock'.

In Milgram's initial studies, 65 per cent of subjects

went all the way up to 450 volts. This was considerably higher than the level of 120–135 volts predicted by a group of psychiatrists before the study began.[40] No one expected ordinary people to continue to 'shock' their subjects even after the learner's protests resulted, at 300 volts, in a refusal to answer further questions. Despite several decades of criticism by his colleagues – mostly on ethical grounds – Milgram's experiment continues to fascinate and perturb us equally. The person must be a rare one who hasn't asked themselves, on hearing of the experiment, 'How far would *I* go?' Milgram's results seemed to turn the ideals of normal society upside down.

Take middle-class housewife Elinor Rosenblum, for example.* A university graduate, Mrs Rosenblum had thrown herself into public life. She volunteered as a mentor for school dropouts, helped with Girl Scouts and was active in the parent–teacher association. Her teenage daughter was an honours student. Yet Mrs Rosenblum made it to the end of the board, twice delivering a shock of 450 volts to the learner. 'It is almost as if she were two women,' Milgram reflected, referring to the difference between the 'competent public performance' Mrs Rosenblum presented to the learner and the agitation she showed to the experimenter.[41]

Was Mrs Rosenblum normal, despite behaving in a way that appeared to conflict with her values? Post-war

* A pseudonym chosen by Milgram, like all names used in the study. One wonders if the one Milgram used for the deceptive veneer of this perfect, all-American woman – Elinor Rosenblum – was intentionally similar to Ethel Rosenberg, the unremarkable and respectable middle-class housewife who was sensationally arrested and found guilty of being a Soviet agent in 1951, and executed, along with her husband Julian, in 1953.

commentators saw the Milgram experiment as evidence of the dangers of conformity, linking it to Nazi Germany or a Cold War fear of communism. 'If Hitler asked you to electrocute a stranger, would you?' asked *Esquire* magazine in 1963, concluding, 'Probably.'[42] The solution was ever greater individualism – or was it? Maybe an individualistic life bred isolation and the breakdown of communities, as implicated in the murder of a young Italian American woman named Catherine Susan Genovese (Kitty, as newspapers called her) in the early hours of 13 March 1964. 'For more than half an hour,' *The New York Times* reported on 27 March, two weeks after Genovese's death, '38 respectable, law-abiding citizens in Queens watched a killer stalk and stab a woman in three separate attacks in Kew Gardens.'[43] These thirty-eight normal people became the stuff of legend, a myth of urban apathy – even if the number of actual witnesses was never really confirmed, and two of them did actually call the police after all.[44]

By the mid-twentieth century, normal society had become a matter of concern as much as one of celebration. What was normal was not necessarily desirable. Or was this in part because normal standards were themselves changing? When Genovese's girlfriend, Mary Ann Zielonko, identified her partner's body, she was subjected to hours of questioning by the police, including a highly inappropriate request to know 'what lesbians did in bed'.[45] The implication was that Genovese's lifestyle was in some way to blame for her death. Who, then, was ultimately normal? The 'apathetic' bystanders, or the popular young bar manager and her live-in girlfriend? This question threads through a surprising number of late twentieth-century stories, unacknowledged and often invisible, but there nonetheless when we stop to look for it.

'What is normal today will no longer be so tomorrow, and vice versa,' Émile Durkheim reflected. 'What is morbid for individuals may be normal for society.'[46] It is only when we seek out the insidious hidden 'normal' that we can see the ways in which social change has worked to support the status quo. The way normal society has been constructed in the industrial West, like the way the normal person has been, is at odds with the reality of not just how *some* people live, but how *most* people live. When marketing consultant Kevin O'Keefe decided to begin a search for the 'average American' in the early 2000s, he quickly discovered that assumptions about what was ordinary did not necessarily align with averages. The most typical American was not, after all, someone living in a heterosexual nuclear family, which made up only a quarter of American homes. 'Families consisting of a working dad, stay-at-home mom, and offspring' – the quintessential Middletown stereotype – made up a mere 7 per cent of homes in the 2000 census.[47]

This gap, between what is average or usual and what we consider as normal or ordinary, highlights the way in which the normal has been intentionally and unconsciously shaped through history. Just as the Harvard Grant Study originally aimed to not only identify the leaders of the future but shape a society in their image, so too do assumptions about normal society continue to affect the ways we think and behave, the running of our institutions and our legal and civil structures. The entire legal framework in England is peppered with terms like 'reasonable', only ever defined in reference to the beliefs of a hypothetical average person. The 'Miller Test' of the US Supreme Court has, since 1973, similarly referred to the beliefs of 'the average person, applying contemporary community standards' in making obscenity judgments. While both systems recognise that normal standards change, they do not doubt that an average, reasonable or 'normal' person exists in any given era. But who is this person, the so-called 'man on the Clapham omnibus'? As we have seen throughout this book, he (or she or they) doesn't actually exist.

THE NEW NORMAL?

Where does all this leave us, in the 'new normal'? I neared the end of this book as much of Britain began the move out of lockdown, in spring 2021. Everyone I spoke to about it was torn, between a desire for things to go 'back to normal' and fear of what this might mean. An early optimism born of mutual aid and community cohesion had seemingly collapsed into a divided world of online consumerism for some home-workers versus food banks and welfare battles for the less fortunate. For decades, certain things had been taken for granted – the legal system, a state education, healthcare, work and the nine-to-five day, and increasing rents and housing prices. In such an apparently stable world, society appeared to simply exist, an unchanging and unchangeable force surrounding its inhabitants. The assumption that this is true is as often made by those who are disenfranchised by normative expectations as for those who benefit from them. The education we receive, the homes we live in, the work we do and the hours we keep are governed by our ideas of what's normal just as much as our attitudes to race, gender, sexuality or immigration.

How often do we fail to spot these preconceived notions about what's normal, threaded as they are through everything we say and do, throughout the world around us? As a teenager, I desperately wanted to have a regional accent (probably Mancunian, or South Wales at a push), because I thought I didn't have one. Some years back, an American friend commented on my Kentish accent. When I protested that I didn't have one, he pointed out that I have a tendency to say 'I' as 'Oi'. I – or should that be Oi – sometimes notice myself doing it now. But before he commented on it, I just thought I sounded like 'everyone else'. But who was that 'everyone' anyway? A decade earlier, it might have been the cut-glass RP (received pronunciation) accents on the nation's televisions, which foreign actors still tend to emulate if they want to sound British. By the 1990s, most people in the south-east, like me, spoke a more informal Estuary English. Neither was a national majority, even if you might be misled into thinking so since both now tend to dominate on TV. Yet to me, the way I spoke had been unquestionably normal. People only had an accent if they sounded different from me.

Sometimes, then, we notice the normal standards in society only when we spot others who are different from our expectations. We are perhaps more likely to notice the norms themselves when they conflict with our own beliefs and lifestyles. The rest of the time, however, what we see is just so usual, so expected, that we don't even notice it at all. Yet this invisible normal has its own history. And the history of normal society is even shorter than that of the normal or average person. In the late nineteenth century scientists, doctors and philosophers – the new 'average men' – came to assume that the same laws applied to the social organism as to the species. This meant that late Victorian society became, to these men, a natural state of affairs: it was normal for wealth and power to be concentrated in the hands of a few. A handful of white, Western, capitalist societies, meanwhile, became representative of the rest of the world, enforcing their norms on to other cultures through a colonial legacy whose impacts are felt into the present day.

Yet even when the lens was turned on the West itself, as in Middletown, a process of exclusion and emphasis continued to select certain people to stand in for society. In 1920s Muncie, this was middle-class white America. Rather than interrogating 'normal' life, Middletown served to reinforce – or create – the idea of a normal society based only on a chosen few. The study also, however, shows how the very meaning of normal has twisted and changed. Normal, in Middletown, was sometimes the statistical average. Sometimes it was the practice or custom that was most common. And, in the book's public reception, the normal was commonly thought of as an ideal, based on those who were thought to be the best of the town's citizens (whether they were members of the Ku Klux Klan or not). The normal was something to be expected or aspired to. It's this last meaning that was also applied to young men participating in the Harvard Grant Study in 1938, along with the notion that to be 'normal' meant to be in good physical and mental health.

In part it's the complex set of meanings behind the word normal that have allowed it to maintain such a hold on us over time. Normal can be almost whatever you want it to be. It can apply to the everyday, the mundane and the monotonous, but also be an ideal or an expectation. Ultimately, however, its history makes it clear that social norms are not discrete entities that miraculously come into existence as part of a living, breathing social organism (whatever Herbert Spencer would have had us believe). Norms emerge from – and are used to support – particular ideological platforms.

What can we do about this difficult and often unpleasant history? It is important, of course, for us to recognise the way definitions of normal have excluded as much as they included: Black people, working-class people, immigrants, inner-city dwellers and rural communities did not fit the Middletown ideal. More than that, however, we need to interrogate and reveal the blank space at the centre. We should ask what normality means in a particular context and how it has been constituted. For Durkheim, 'social facts' had to be useful, but what uses have these norms performed? They have propped up hierarchies – evolutionary or economic – and benefitted some at the expense of others. Yet the structures of today's society are no more natural and inevitable than the colonialist policies of Herbert Spencer's time. If we have learned anything from the Covid-19 pandemic, let it be to question if we should be seeking a new normal at all.

EPILOGUE
BEYOND THE NORMAL

I have a clear memory of standing at a bus stop, somewhere on the North Circular Road in London, aged about twenty-one. It was late, and the headlights shone through the chill night air as each car whipped past with a mechanical snarl. The street was far above, hidden from view behind the shrubs that huddled along the dimly lit, zigzag path. I would never have walked down to that bus stop alone.

But I wasn't alone that night. My boyfriend was with me, hands stuffed into his pockets, stamping his feet impatiently in the graffitied bus shelter that gave little respite from the winter wind. In those days, when mobile phones didn't yet have cameras let alone the internet, you never knew how long you'd have to wait for a bus. Cold and bored, I began to dance to warm up. I may even have started singing. My boyfriend glowered at me. 'Why can't I just have a *normal* girlfriend?' he complained.

What did he mean by normal? He probably didn't really know himself. His words were certainly intended as an insult: he was tired, cold and moody, and he may also have been fed up with the recurring dramas associated with my not-very-stable mental health. In retrospect I can see that this was stressful and draining for him, though at the time I don't think I appreciated this. His words were also an effort to get me to change my behaviour, to fit in with some perceived ideal, even if neither of us knew quite what that was. Some years later, two of my housemates spent the entire journey back from a club arguing over which of them could claim the honour of being the sole normal person in our group. 'None of us are normal,' the two of us who hadn't bothered to try to win the title objected. 'That's why we're friends!'

In everyday life, it often seems like common sense to judge what's normal or desirable based on our own experiences, just as we have seen white, wealthy men do time and time again throughout history. Yet not only are we all coming from different perspectives and backgrounds, and rarely have a clear idea of what we mean by normal anyway, but our life experiences are also formed in relation to historically created expectations about what's normal. These are embedded in our daily lives, in our institutions, medical practices, politics and international relations. They affect us whether we meet the 'norm' or not.

My idea of what's normal is shaped by growing up as a white, middle-class girl in suburban southern England, and all the opportunities that gave me, as well as the recognition of difference formed from being a not-so-wealthy child in a selective state school full of very privileged youngsters. My fears about not being normal were formed despite the fact I have often benefitted from my proximity to the average man championed by the Victorians. When we criticise the normal as a historical category we have to unpick the way it is bound into our lives, from birth to death. That's why the personal anecdotes are an important part of this book whether you, as a reader, identify with them or have had very different experiences. They too demand questioning and comparison.

As we come to the end of our journey through the history of the normal, we have seen this failure to question occur time and time again. We are aware that the normal as a category is not simply an average or a representation of nature but something that has been constructed, in medicine, science and popular culture, from Quetelet's 'average man' to the Harvard Grant Study of 'normal' young men. Almost every incarnation of the normal shares a set of characteristics. In the West, to be 'normal' is to be white, male, middle class, able-bodied, cisgendered and heterosexual. That this is not the same as being statistically average is clear from the fact that these attributes are rarely the most common in any population. In 1920s Middletown, for example, white, middle-class men formed at most 15 per cent of the population.

Like the measurements of Norma, typical woman, which turned out not to describe any one individual at all, this 'normal' fits far fewer people than we might anticipate. A recent online course I took for work asked me to give my answers to just six personal characteristics, including age, gender and marital status, comparing them to statistical data for the entire country from the 2011 census. My answers, it told me, are shared with a mere half a million people in the UK: less than 1 per cent of the population. The idea that some majority group exists that personifies the so-called normal is an illusion. Nor is there any inherent value in presumed 'normal' traits. It is simply the case that those possessing them have, throughout much of the history we have explored, happened to be the people that held power.

It is perhaps easiest to recognise the existence of a particular definition of normal when you have been excluded from it in one way or another. From the 1830s to the 1960s and well beyond, the countless people not reflected by the 'average man' have been doubly excluded. First, they were removed from the data that created the averages: Middletown and Kinsey excluded African Americans, for example, while Galton and his colleagues altered female data to fit male measurements. Then, these people were found not to meet the normal ideal generated from these averages. Despite this exclusion, prescriptive notions of normality based on race, class, gender and sexuality have been used as a guide for the lives and behaviour of all citizens in countries across Europe, North America and beyond. The normal became an expected achievement, rather than a measure of variation, an ideal to be attained whether you want – and are able – to or not.

There are considerable consequences to this, even today in our modern world. Those who do not meet predefined norms may be punitively sanctioned. They may be labelled as different, as criminals or mentally ill. They may be locked up in prisons or psychiatric hospitals, denied state support or healthcare. Entire communities may find themselves cruelly segregated. The widespread practice of racial segregation, whereby schools, housing, transport and countless other elements of daily life were forcibly separated depending on whether one happened to be black or white, was legally ended in the US with the Civil Rights Act of 1964. Yet, in many cities and many countries, a separation of citizens by race and class continues to this day, compounded by poverty and social inequality.

Difference is not always punished, of course. Sometimes it may simply be erased, in support of the mistaken notion that 'normal' is a majority status, just as newspapers in the 1960s erased Kitty Genovese's lesbian identity so completely it was a full fifty years before a researcher would restore it to the public image of her life.[1] Or, to use a contemporary example, take the controversy surrounding deadnaming – using the birth or pre-transition name of a trans person. This disrespect is damaging on an individual level, of course, causing distress and harming relationships; on a wider level, this practice plays into the notion that there is a certain kind of normal and those who do not or cannot conform to it can be forced to do so by delegitimising their difference.

While this seems to have been largely forgotten today, in the 1960s the normal came into open question in medicine, science, philosophy and popular thought. It was also, paradoxically, increasingly discussed. In Britain, North America and Europe physicians debated whether the normal child existed, and tried to define normal health, weight and blood pressure. Psychologists studied the reactions of 'normal' people to unpleasant situations or their willingness to follow orders. Average or usual behaviour was not, people newly worried, necessarily desirable or even possible. Yet, by discussing the normal like never before, these post-war studies continued to support the idea that some kind of average or usual behaviour existed, if only we could find and understand it.

One reason that the power of the normal remains strong is because it has often been defined by its opposite: the so-called abnormal. The average man was cast as the centre of gravity in society, 'around which oscillate the social elements'.[2] This implied that the normal was unchanging, monolithic, a kind of fixed entity that supported all other variation. The normal began as both average and ideal and, because it was also fictitious, it was easy to understand it as the status quo, the wealthy white men at the centre of the universe. Their position was fixed largely because they created the normal in their image, by judging all other human beings in comparison to themselves. The normal standard is a belief system, an illusion that infiltrates the entirety of modern Western society. No one is Norma, typical woman. No one is Quetelet's average man. Yet the normal remains a bit like the Emperor's new clothes: something we might want to question but are too embarrassed or uncertain to refute entirely.

While writing this book, I learned a great deal about how easy it is to reproduce normative judgements without even realising. There were points where I unthinkingly allowed the norms I had grown up with to go unchallenged, where I unwittingly reproduced binary ways of thinking or value judgements. There probably still are, despite the ruthless attentions of critical friends. In our desire for straightforward and coherent explanations for existence we may try to force a square peg into a round hole just to proceed along a linear narrative. Yet 'the world is not to be divided into sheep and goats', as Kinsey memorably put it.

There will undoubtedly be things that have touched your life that I could have included in these pages and didn't. But this is, I hope, just the beginning of the story, and there are countless more tales that require telling. The way we tell them is as important as the stories themselves. Our assumptions about the categories of normal and abnormal have long given us a convenient way of arranging a narrative which, sometimes, we accept without thinking because it's the easier path. I hope that, the next time you find yourself at such a crossroads, this book reminds you to question your journey and consider how else it might be approached.

I leave you, finally, to think about how the very questions we ask shape the way we think and feel about normality. In Douglas Adams's *The Hitchhiker's Guide to the Galaxy*, a super-computer named Deep Thought takes 7.5 million years to calculate the answer to life, the universe and everything as a pleasingly simplistic 42. But this only reveals that no one knows what the ultimate *question* of life, the universe and everything is. Questions, in real life as in science fiction, are just as important as answers, sometimes more so.

Am I normal, then? Well, yes and no. But is that, ultimately, the right question to ask?

ACKNOWLEDGEMENTS

When I told my god-daughter Willow, then aged eleven, the subject of the new book I was writing she expressed a certain amount of disbelief before offering to write it for me. The folded piece of A4 paper she produced took pride of place on my desk and has kept me going in the three long years since. 'Am I normal?' asks the cover of Willow's book and the question is answered inside: 'NO! Deal with it.' It's a beautiful summary of a complicated topic.

There are many other people I'd like to thank for their help in the writing of this book, and the research on which it has been built. I could not have done any of it without all the archives and libraries I've used: the Wellcome Library, the British Library, the Royal College of Nursing Library and Archive, the archive of the Royal Academy of Science, Letters and Fine Arts of Belgium, UCL Special Collections, the Salvation Army International Heritage Centre and Bethlem Museum of the Mind. Especial thanks are due to Ross MacFarlane and Alice White at the Wellcome Library for their ideas and suggestions and Subhadra Das and Hannah Cornish at UCL for talking me through the Galton Collection.

My thanks are also due to my colleagues at Queen Mary, University of London and the Royal College of Nursing who have supported me through this work, in particular Anna Semmens at the RCN and Thomas Dixon at QMUL, who have been unfailingly supportive managers, and Emma Sutton and Frances Reed, who offered their time to read and discuss early drafts and final chapters. I would also like to thank the other friends, family members and colleagues who kindly read draft chapters and offered useful suggestions and criticisms: Åsa Jansson, Debbie Shipton, Becky Matthews, Indy Lalli, Lauren Cracknell, Alice Nicholls, Sasha Garwood Lloyd, Sally Frampton, Gemma Angel, Gail Robertson, Shaz Lockwood, Nat Hayden, Tara and Mike Alexander, Jane Fradgley, Brian and Kathy Chaney, Alison Feeney and Stewart Caine.

An enormous debt of gratitude is owed to Francesca Barrie, my editor, for her advice, criticism and enthusiasm throughout. This book is much better because of her. Thanks also to everyone at Wellcome and Profile Books, in particular Sam Matthews for copy-editing, and to the Wellcome Trust for funding much of the research on which this book is based.

Writing in isolation can be a soul-destroying process, and I'm incredibly grateful to everyone who has kept me going. Thanks to the Post Doc crew at QMUL for those invaluable weekly catchups, and to the Ministry of Fun at the RCN for crosswords and quizzes. Thanks to Michelle, Sadie (Queen of Quiplash) and Willow (Queen of Gotham) for virtual games and vegan treats, and to Kate, Lee-Anne and Sheila for watch-alongs from afar. And a massive thank you to the Genting gang, who I've been lucky enough to see more than ever in the last couple of years: Gail, Shaz, Nat, Tara and Holly, love you for ever.

Last but very much not least, thank you to my family for their unfailing support. To Stewart, who read and compared repeated drafts with remarkably little complaint (and to Charles and Erik the cats, who provided much-needed cuddles). To Mum and Dad for their suggestions and interest, and to Ali for the most incredibly thoughtful comments on chapter 6, and for getting me out of London on all-too-rare occasions.

And finally, much love to the newest members of the family: to Annabel, with whom online baking has been a real highlight of the past two years, and to Lara, whose infectious smile stays with me always.

CHARTS AND
QUESTIONNAIRES

273 International Health Exhibition Anthropometric Laboratory card, from Francis Galton, *Anthropometric Laboratory*, 1884

274 Search-for-Norma Entry form, *Cleveland Plain Dealer*, 9 September 1945

275 Census of Hallucinations, 1889, from 'Report on the Census of Hallucinations', *Proceedings of the Society for Psychical Research* 10 (1894), Appendix A

276 Personality Schedule, from L. L. Thurstone and Thelma Gwinn Thurstone, 'A Neurotic Inventory', *Journal of Social Psychology* 1, no. 1 (1930)
For answers, see page 283

277 Masculinity–Femininity Test / Attitude–Interest Analysis Test, from Lewis M. Terman and Catharine Cox Miles, *Sex and Personality*, 1936
For answers, see page 284

278 Mass Observation Questionnaire on Sexual Behaviour, 28 March 1949

279 A Scale of Emotional Maturity, 1931, from R. R. Willoughby, 'A Scale of Emotional Maturity', *Journal of Social Psychology* 3, no. 1 (1932)

280 The Empathy Test: Form A, by Willard A. Kerr, 1947

281 Binet–Simon Intelligence Test: Problem Solving, 1905, from Alfred Binet and Théodore Simon, *The Development of Intelligence in Children*, 1916
For answers, see page 284

282 Army Alpha IQ Test, from Clarence Yoakum and Robert Yerkes, *Army Mental Tests*, 1920
For answers, see page 284

INTERNATIONAL HEALTH EXHIBITION, 1884

ANTHROPOMETRIC LABORATORY,

Arranged by FRANCIS GALTON, F.R.S.

Age last birthday? ——————————————

Married or unmarried? ——————————————

Birthplace? ——————————————

Occupation? ——————————————

Residence in town, suburb or country? ——————————————

Sex ——————— Colour of eyes ———————

Date ——————— Initials ———————

EYESIGHT

	right eye	left eye
Greatest distance in inches, of reading "Diamond" type }		

Colour sense, good-ness of }

JUDGMENT OF EYE

	in three parts	in two parts
Error per cent, in dividing a line of 15 inches }		

Error in degrees of estimating squareness }

HEARING

Keenness can hardly be tested here owing to the noises and echoes.

Highest note audible }	between	0.000 and 0.000	vibrations per second.

SWIFTNESS

of blow of hand in feet per second } ——— ——— feet per second

STRENGTH

squeeze in lbs. of } right hand ——— of pull in lbs.
left " }

SPAN OF ARMS

From finger tips of opposite hands } ——— feet, ——— inches.

HEIGHT

Sitting, measured from seat of chair } ——— feet, ——— inches.

Standing in shoes ——— feet, ——— inches.

less height of heel.............. ——— inches.

Height without shoes ——— feet, ——— inches.

WEIGHT

In ordinary in-door clothing in lbs. } ———

BREATHING POWER

Greatest expiration in cubic inches } ———

SEARCH-FOR-NORMA ENTRY

Norma Editor: Please enter my dimensions as given below in the "Search for Norma:"

NAME _____

ADDRESS _____

CITY _____ ZONE ____

OCCUPATION _____

AGE _____ SINGLE or MARRIED   Number of CHILDREN ____
                (circle which)

Dimensions Table in Inches and Pounds

HEIGHT	58	59	60	61	62	63	64	65	66	67	68
	58½	59½	60½	61½	62½	63½	64½	65½	66½	67½	68½
BUST	30	31	32	33	34	35	36	37	38	39	40
	30½	31½	32½	33½	34½	35½	36½	37½	38½	39½	40½
WAIST	25	26	27	28	29	30	31	32	33	34	35
	25½	26½	27½	28½	29½	30½	31½	32½	33½	34½	35½
HIPS	34	35	36	37	38	39	40	41	42	43	44
	34½	35½	36½	37½	38½	39½	40½	41½	42½	43½	44½
THIGH	15	16	17	18	19	20	21	22	23	24	25
	15½	16½	17½	18½	19½	20½	21½	22½	23½	24½	25½
CALF	10	10½	11	11½	12	12½	13	13½	14	14½	15
ANKLE	8¼	8½	8¾	9	9¼	9½	9¾	10	10¼	10½	10¾
FOOT	7¾	8	8¼	8½	8¾	9	9¼	9½	9¾	10	10¼
WEIGHT	118	120	122	124	126	128	130	132	134	136	138
	119	121	123	125	127	129	131	133	135	137	139

INSTRUCTIONS:

MEASURE bust at the fullest point, waist at the narrowest, hips at the top of the bone just below the waist, thigh midway between hip bone and knee joint, calf at the fullest when the foot is flat, ankle on the inside bulge, foot (right) from heel to big toe with the foot flat. Keep your tape parallel to the floor in all measurements.

MARK your dimensions, using nearest number, on the table above by blacking out the blocks containing each of your dimensions.

MAIL ENTRY at once to Norma Editor, 508 Plain Dealer Building, Cleveland 16, O., using this coupon or exact facsimile.

Cleveland Plain Dealer, 9 Sept. 1945

Census of Hallucinations, 1889.

☞ Please return this paper when filled up to
PROFESSOR SIDGWICK,
Cambridge.

B *International Congress of Experimental Psychology.*

FURTHER ANSWERS TO BE ADDRESSED TO ANY PERSON ANSWERING YES TO THE QUESTION OF SCHEDULE A. Namely:—Have you ever, when believing yourself to be completely awake, had a vivid impression of seeing, or being touched by a living being, or inanimate object, or of hearing a voice; which impression, so far as you could discover, was not due to any external physical cause?

1. Please state what you saw or heard or felt, and give the place, date and hour of the experience as nearly as you can.

2. How were you occupied at the time, and were you out of health or in grief or anxiety? What was your age?

3. Was the impression that of someone whom you were in the habit of seeing, and do you know what he or she was doing at the time?

4. Were there other persons present with you at the time, and if so did they in any way share the experience?

5. Please state whether you have had such an experience more than once, and if so give particulars of the different occasions.

6. Any notes taken at the time, or other information about the experiences will be gratefully received.

Signature _____

Address _____

Date _____

No names or addresses will be published without special permission.

From the Psychological Laboratory of the University of Chicago.

PERSONALITY SCHEDULE

1928 Edition

Name ....

      (Last Name)   (Given Names or Initials)

The questions in this blank are intended to indicate various emotional and personality traits. Your answers may reveal a well-adjusted emotional life or they may show that you have some form of nervousness or worry which you may not yourself understand completely.

In front of each question you will find: yes no ?

Draw a ring around one of these three answers for each question. Try to answer by "yes" or "no" if it is possible.

1b-1	Do you laugh easily?	yes	no	?
1b-2	Do you worry too long over humiliating experiences?	yes	no	?
1b-3	Are you careful not to say things to hurt people's feeling?	yes	no	?
1b-4	Are you sometimes the leader at a social affair?	yes	no	?
1b-5	Are your day-dreams about improbable occurrences?	yes	no	?
1b-7	Do you usually get turned around in new places?	yes	no	?
1b-8	Do you often feel lonesome, even when you are with other people?	yes	no	?
1b-9	Do you love your father more than your mother?	yes	no	?
1b-10	Do you consider yourself a rather nervous person?	yes	no	?
1b-11	Are you afraid of falling when you are on a high place?	yes	no	?
1b-13	Are you interested in meeting a lot of different kinds of people?	yes	no	?
1b-15	Do a great many things frighten you?	yes	no	?
1b-16	Have you ever had a nervous breakdown?	yes	no	?
1b-17	Are your feelings easily hurt?	yes	no	?
1b-18	Are you easily shocked by sexual topics, *risqué* stories, and the like?	yes	no	?
1b-19	Do you keep in the background on social occasions?	yes	no	?

For answers, see page 283

You are asked to cooperate seriously and carefully in marking the items in this booklet. This is not an intelligence test. We want to find out something about the attitudes and interests of people in relation to their occupations, their home situations, and their hobbies.

Name .... Age .... Sex .... Race ....
City .... State ....
Underline one: Single, Married, Widowed, Separated, Divorced.

EXERCISE 2

Directions:— Here are some drawings, a little like ink blots. They are not pictures of anything in particular but might suggest almost anything to you, just as shapes in the clouds sometimes do. Beside each drawing four things are mentioned. Underline the one word that tells what the drawing makes you think of most.

Examples:—

baby
dog
man
squirrel

arm
flame
flower
tail

dog's head
glove
hand
horse's head

			Omission
1.	jar	0	0
	mail box	–	
	pipe	+	
	tombstone	+	
2.	ball bat	–	0
	ham	0	
	pear	+	
	tadpole	+	
3.	candle	0	0
	cup	0	
	hat	+	
	inkwell	–	
4.	fish	0	0
	mirror	0	
	snow shoe	+	
	spoon	–	

FROM LEWIS M. TERMAN AND CATHARINE COX
MILES, *SEX AND PERSONALITY*, 1936

For answers, see page 284

| a) Sex |
| b) Age |
| c) Age at which full-time education ceased |

20a Are you, or have you been, engaged
    to be married? (Say which) _____
  b IF NOT NOW ENGAGED - Have you any
    particular man/woman friend at
    present? _____
  c IF NO TO b - Have you ever had a
    particular man/woman friend?

21a Have you ever had sexual intercourse
    with any man/woman?   Yes... No...
  b IF YES - When did you last have
    intercourse with any man/woman?

22a Have you ever gone in for love-making
    which stopped short only of intercourse? Yes... No...
  b IF YES - How usual has it been for you
    to experience a sexual climax in this
    sort of love-making?

25a With how many different men/women
    have you had sexual intercourse?
  b Were you in love with this person/
    any of these people?
  c IF ENGAGED - Have you had sexual
    intercourse with your fiancé(e)?

31a Have you ever had sex relations with
    anyone of the same sex as yourself?   Yes... No...
  b NO TO a - Have you gone in for any
    sort of love-making with anyone of the
    same sex as yourself?
  c IF YES TO a or b - When did this last occur?
    During last year.. last 5 years.. 10 years.. 20 years.. Longer..
  d IF YES TO a or b - How usual has it been
    for you to experience a sexual climax
    in these relationships?

32a Do you ever experience any sort of sexual
    pleasure in dreams at night?   Yes... No...
  b IF YES TO a - When did this last occur?
  c IF YES TO a - How usual is it for you to
    experience a sexual climax when you have
    these dreams at night?

33a Have you ever masturbated?   Yes... No...
  b IF YES TO a - When did you last masturbate?
  c IF YES TO a - How usual is it for you to
    experience a sexual climax when you masturbate?
  d IF YES TO a - How usual is it for you to have
    some sort of day-dream or fantasy when you
    masturbate?
  e IF HAVE DAY-DREAM - Very roughly, what does
    this day-dream usually consist of?

36a On the whole, would you say that you yourself are sexually
    normal, or not? IF NOT -
  b In what ways do you think you may not be sexually normal?

A SCALE OF EMOTIONAL MATURITY, 1931

'*S*' in each of the following situations is, for the moment, your subject. If the subject's reaction in a situation much like that described was (a) similar to the one described, circle the 3; (b) different from the one described, circle the 0. If you have never encountered the subject in a situation like that described, but believe that his reaction to it would be (a) similar to the one described, circle the 2; (b) different from the one described, circle the 1. Complete the scale for yourself and ask two friends, relatives or colleagues to score you as a subject. A higher score on the test denotes greater emotional maturity.

1.	*S* is ordinarily friendly toward members of his immediate social group, but in critical periods becomes irritable and hostile.	0	1	2	3
6.	*S* is extremely solicitous of his immediate family associates.	0	1	2	3
7.	*S* makes his plans with objective reference to his own death when this issue is involved; no emotional reaction involved greater than that, for instance, concerned in planning with reference to a long journey.	0	1	2	3
9.	*S* is meticulous in matters of dress; a considerable part of his income is spent in this activity, even though strict economies are thereby necessitated elsewhere.	0	1	2	3
10.	*S* chooses courses of action with reference to his own maximum immediate satisfaction.	0	1	2	3
11.	*S* develops affective difficulty in the presence of a necessity for precise or realistic thinking, e.g., mathematics.	0	1	2	3
12.	*S* is faced with an instance of violation of his mores; he is intellectually interested, without emotional shock, and seeks to discover what motives and satisfaction are involved from the standpoint of the violator.	0	1	2	3
15.	*S* is deprived of a much anticipated opportunity; he redoubles his efforts to gain just this objective.	0	1	2	3
17.	*S* characteristically appeals for help in the solution of his problems.	0	1	2	3
23.	*S* is rather self-conscious in the presence of individuals of markedly greater prestige than his own.	0	1	2	3
25.	*S* conducts himself in discussion as if the only objective of the discussion were the mutual discovery of truth.	0	1	2	3
26.	When driving an automobile, *S* is unperturbed in ordinary situations, but becomes angry with other drivers who impede his progress.	0	1	2	3
29.	*S*'s day-dreams represent the reversal of situations humiliating in the real world.	0	1	2	3
31.	*S* believes in democracy in principle, but prefers not to associate too closely with individuals from groups widely divergent from his own.	0	1	2	3
34.	*S* demands that he be punctiliously served in hotels, sleeping cars, etc.	0	1	2	3

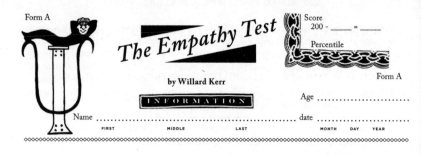

Form A

The Empathy Test

by Willard Kerr

INFORMATION

Score
200 - _____ = _____
Percentile

Form A

Age ....

Name .... date ....
FIRST   MIDDLE   LAST   MONTH   DAY   YEAR

DIRECTIONS

How well do you know the likes and dislikes of average people? In ALL these test items try to place yourself in the position of the hypothetical average person. Answer the questions NOT AS YOU but as the average person would answer.

1. What music does the average non-office FACTORY WORK-ER prefer at work? Rank these types in order of their probable popularity among the non-office factory workers of the United States. Assign a rank of "1" to the most popular, "2" to the second most popular, etc., and "14" to the least popular.

RANK	MUSIC
____	polkas
____	classical
____	waltzes
____	fast dance
____	western
____	sacred
____	"Hit Parade" type
____	hill billy
____	semi-classical
____	spirituals
____	Hawaiian
____	square dances
____	humor-novelty
____	blues

•••••••••••••• (fold here when you have finished the test) ••••••••••••••

2. What does the average American choose to read? Rank these magazines in order from most to least TOTAL PAID CIRCULATION.

RANK	MAGAZINE
____	Prairie Farmer
____	Silver Screen
____	Reader's Digest
____	Popular Mechanics
____	Saturday Evening Post
____	Good Housekeeping
____	Esquire
____	Atlantic Monthly
____	United States News
____	Fortune
____	Parents' Magazine
____	Antiques
____	Ladies' Home Journal
____	National Geographic
____	New Republic

3. Here are ten commonly annoying experiences to PERSONS AGED 25-39. Imagine yourself the AVERAGE PERSON of this age level and rank from most to least annoying the following.

RANK	ANNOYING EXPERIENCE
____	A boisterous person attracting attention
____	Hearing a person chewing gum
____	Seeing a person's nose running
____	A person coughing in my face
____	A person slapping me on the back
____	A person constantly trying to be funny
____	A person using a great deal of slang
____	A person monopolizing conversation
____	The odor of bad breath
____	Being told to do something just as I am about to do it

Most children aged 15 should be able to solve these tests correctly. A correct response to each question is required.

1. A woman walking in the forest of Fontainebleau stopped suddenly dreadfully frightened, hurried to the nearest policeman and told him that she had just seen hanging to the limb of a tree _____ (after a pause) what?

2. My neighbour has just received some singular visitors. He received one after the other a doctor, a lawyer and a priest. What is going on at my neighbour's?

For answers, see page 284

ARMY ALPHA IQ TEST, 1920

Notice the sample sentence:

People **hear** with the   eyes   <u>ears</u>   nose   mouth

The correct word is **ears**, because it makes the truest sentence.

In each of the sentences below you have four choices for the last word. Only one of them is correct. In each sentence draw a line under the one of these four words which makes the truest sentence. If you cannot be sure, guess. The two samples are already marked as they should be.

SAMPLES $\left\{ \begin{array}{l} \text{People } \textbf{hear} \text{ with the} \quad \text{eyes} \quad \underline{\text{ears}} \quad \text{nose} \quad \text{mouth} \\ \text{France is in } \quad \underline{\text{Europe}} \quad \text{Asia} \quad \text{Africa} \quad \text{Australia} \end{array} \right.$

1   **America** was discovered by   Drake   Hudson   Columbus   Balboa 1

2   **Pinochle** is played with   rackets   cards   pins   dice 2

3   The most prominent industry in **Detroit** is   automobiles   brewing   flour   packing 3

4   The **Wyandotte** is a kind of   horse   fowl   cattle   granite 4

5   The **U. S. School for Army Officers** is at   Annapolis   West Point   New Haven   Ithaca 5

6   **Food products** are made by   Smith & Wesson   Swift & Co.   W. L. Douglas   B. T. Babbitt 6

7   **Bud Fisher** is famous as an   actor   author   baseball player   comic artist 7

8   The **Guernsey** is a kind of   horse   goat   sheep   cow 8

9   **Marguerite Clark** is known as a   suffragist   singer   movie actress   writer 9

10 **"Hasn't scratched yet"** is used in advertising a   duster   flour   brush   cleanser 10

For answers, see page 284

282

ANSWERS

From the *Psychological Laboratory of the University of Chicago.*

PERSONALITY SCHEDULE ANSWERS

1928 Edition

Neurotic answer

1b-1	Do you laugh easily?	No
1b-2	Do you worry too long over humiliating experiences?	Yes
1b-3	Are you careful not to say things to hurt people's feeling?	No
1b-4	Are you sometimes the leader at a social affair?	No
1b-5	Are your day-dreams about improbable occurrences?	Yes
1b-7	Do you usually get turned around in new places?	Yes
1b-8	Do you often feel lonesome, even when you are with other people?	Yes
1b-9	Do you love your father more than your mother?	Yes
1b-10	Do you consider yourself a rather nervous person?	Yes
1b-11	Are you afraid of falling when you are on a high place?	Yes
1b-13	Are you interested in meeting a lot of different kinds of people?	No
1b-15	Do a great many things frighten you?	Yes
1b-16	Have you ever had a nervous breakdown?	Yes, ?
1b-17	Are your feelings easily hurt?	Yes
1b-18	Are you easily shocked by sexual topics, *risqué* stories, and the like?	Yes
1b-19	Do you keep in the background on social occasions?	Yes

L.L. THURSTONE AND THELMA GWINN THURSTONE

+ve scores indicate masculine traits and -ve scores indicate feminine traits.

A. EXERCISE 2

Items	Responses				
	a	*b*	*c*	*d*	O^1
(1)	0	-4	+3	+1	0
(2)	-4	0	+1	+3	0
(3)	0	0	+3	-3	0
(4)	0	0	+1	-1	0

BINET–SIMON INTELLIGENCE TEST: PROBLEM SOLVING, 1905
ANSWERS

1. The only correct response, implied by the context is: *a person who has been hanged.*

2. For the second question the correct response is: *He is very ill, he is dying. —Someone is very ill there, dead.*
Incorrect responses: *I do not know.* An erroneous answer often consists in a repetition of the question. *It happens that he has received a doctor and a priest.*

ARMY ALPHA IQ TEST ANSWERS

1	**Columbus**	6	**Swift & Co.**
2	**cards**	7	**comic artist**
3	**automobiles**	8	**cow**
4	**fowl**	9	**movie actress**
5	**West Point**	10	**cleanser**

LIST OF ILLUSTRATIONS

NOTES

Prologue: Am I Normal?

1 Satadru Sen, 'Schools, Athletes and Confrontation: The Student Body in Colonial India', in *Confronting the Body: The Politics of Physicality in Colonial and Post-Colonial India*, ed. James H. Mills and Satadru Sen (London: Anthem Press, 2004), 66–7.

2 'About Us', Bureau of Indian Education (US Department of the Interior), accessed 12 January 2022, www.bie.edu/topic-page/bureau-indian-education.

3 Joseph Henrich, Steven J. Heine, and Ara Norenzayan, 'The Weirdest People in the World?', *Behavioral and Brain Sciences* 33, no. 2–3 (June 2010): 61–83; Michael D. Gurven and Daniel E. Lieberman, 'WEIRD Bodies: Mismatch, Medicine and Missing Diversity', *Evolution and Human Behavior* 41, no. 5 (1 September 2020): 330–40.

4 Kathryn B. H. Clancy and Jenny L. Davis, 'Soylent Is People, and WEIRD Is White: Biological Anthropology, Whiteness, and the Limits of the WEIRD', *Annual Review of Anthropology* 48, no. 1 (21 October 2019): 169–86.

5 Michael Morris, 'Standard White: Dismantling White Normativity', *California Law Review* 104, no. 4 (2016): 958.

6 Alyson J. McGregor, *Sex Matters: How Male-Centric Medicine Endangers Women's Health and What We Can Do About It* (London: Quercus, 2020), 78–9.

7 Henrich, Heine, and Norenzayan, 'The Weirdest People in the World?', 61.

I A Brief History of the Normal

1   Saul Stahl, 'The Evolution of the Normal Distribution', *Mathematics Magazine* 79, no. 2 (2006): 96–113; Donald Teets and Karen Whitehead, 'The Discovery of Ceres: How Gauss Became Famous', *Mathematics Magazine* 72, no. 2 (1999): 83–93.

2   Theodore M. Porter, 'The Mathematics of Society: Variation and Error in Quetelet's Statistics', *The British Journal for the History of Science* 18, no. 1 (1985): 58.

3   Written in French, the original title was *Sur l'homme et le développement de ses facultés, ou Essai de physique sociale*.

4   NatCen Social Research, UCL, *Health Survey for England 2016: Adult health trends*, Health and Social Care Information Centre, accessed 11 May 2022, healthsurvey.hscic.gov.uk/media/63757/HSE2016-Adult-trends.pdf.

5   Mark F. Schilling, Ann E. Watkins, and William Watkins, 'Is Human Height Bimodal?', *The American Statistician* 56, no. 3 (1 August 2002): 223–9.

6   Adolphe Quetelet, *A Treatise on Man and the Development of His Faculties*, trans. Robert Knox (Edinburgh: W. & R. Chambers, 1842), x.

7   Adolphe Quetelet, *Letters Addressed to HRH the Grand Duke of Saxe-Coburg and Gotha, on the Theory of Probabilities, as Applied to the Moral and Political Sciences*, trans. Olinthus Gregory Downes (London: C. & E. Layton, 1849), 93.

8   Quetelet, *Letters*, 90.

9   Quetelet, *Treatise*, v.

10   Martin Kemp, *Leonardo da Vinci: The Marvellous Works of Nature and Man* (Oxford: Oxford University Press, 2007), 22.

11   Alison Matthews David, 'Tailoring and the "Normal" Body in Nineteenth-Century France', in *Histories of the Normal and the Abnormal*, ed. W. Ernst (London: Routledge, 2006), 151.

12   Peter Cryle and Elizabeth Stephens, *Normality: A Critical Genealogy* (Chicago and London: University of Chicago Press, 2017), 3–4.

13   William McDowall, *History of the Burgh of Dumfries* (Edinburgh: A. & C. Black, 1867), 796–805.

14   Ian Hacking, 'Biopower and the Avalanche of Printed Numbers', *Humanities in Society* 5 (1982): 279–95.

15   For more on these developments, see Jean-Guy Prévost and Jean-Pierre Beaud, *Statistics, Public Debate and the State, 1800–1945* (London: Pickering & Chatto, 2012); Alain Desrosières, *The Politics of Large Numbers: A History of Statistical Reasoning*, trans. Camille Naish (Cambridge, MA and London: Harvard University Press, 1998); Theodore M. Porter, *The Rise of Statistical Thinking, 1820–1900* (Princeton: Princeton University Press, 1986); Kevin Donnelly, 'The Other Average Man: Science Workers in Quetelet's Belgium', *History of Science* 52, no. 4 (2014): 401–28.

16 For more on Broussais's theories and practice see Ian Hacking, *The Taming of Chance* (Cambridge: Cambridge University Press, 1990), 160–66; Georges Canguilhem, *The Normal and the Pathological*, trans. Carolyn R. Fawcett (New York: Zone Books, 1989).

17 Quoted in Canguilhem, *The Normal and the Pathological*, 49.

18 Robert G. W. Kirk and Neil Pemberton, *Leech* (London: Reaktion, 2013), 58.

19 Kirk and Pemberton, *Leech*, 58.

20 This section draws on Mary Pickering, *Auguste Comte: An Intellectual Biography*, vol. 1 (Cambridge: Cambridge University Press, 1993).

21 Frederick James Gould, *Auguste Comte* (London: Watts, 1920), 26.

22 For full details see Pickering, *Auguste Comte*, vol. 1.

23 Hacking, *The Taming of Chance*, 167.

24 Female Patient Casebook for 1898 (CB 159), Bethlem Museum of the Mind, entry 125.

25 Female Patient Casebook for 1881 (CB 119), Bethlem Museum of the Mind, entry 93.

26 Daniel Hack Tuke, 'Eccentricity', in *Dictionary of Psychological Medicine*, ed. Daniel Hack Tuke, vol. 1 (London: J. & A. Churchill, 1892), 419–23.

27 Auguste Comte quoted in Canguilhem, *The Normal and the Pathological*, 49.

28 William Corner, *The Story of the 34th Company (Middlesex) Imperial Yeomanry* (London: T. Fisher Unwin, 1902), 1.

29 Corner, *Story of the 34th*, 11.

30 Vanessa Heggie, 'Lies, Damn Lies, and Manchester's Recruiting Statistics: Degeneration as an "Urban Legend" in Victorian and Edwardian Britain', *Journal of the History of Medicine and Allied Sciences* 63, no. 2 (2008): 182.

31 Arnold White, *Efficiency and Empire* (London: Methuen & Co., 1901), 101–2.

32 Charles F. G. Masterman, 'Realities at Home', in *The Heart of the Empire; Discussions of Problems of Modern City Life in England, with an Essay on Imperialism* (London: T. Fisher Unwin, 1907), 8.

33 For more on White and his figures, see Heggie, 'Lies, Damn Lies, and Manchester's Recruiting Statistics', 183–6.

34 William R. Greg, 'On the Failure of "Natural Selection" in the Case of Man', *Fraser's Magazine for Town and Country*, 1868.

35 Charles Darwin, *The Descent of Man, and Selection in Relation to Sex*, vol. 1 (London: John Murray, 1871), 158.

36 Robert Louis Stevenson, *The Strange Case of Dr Jekyll and Mr Hyde* (London: Penguin, 1994), 23.

37 You can explore the maps online here: https://booth.lse.ac.uk/.

38 Judith R. Walkowitz, *City of Dreadful Delight: Narratives of Sexual Danger in Late-Victorian London* (London: Virago, 1992).

39 William H. Kruskal and Stephen M. Stigler, 'Normative Terminology: "Normal" in Statistics and Elsewhere', in *Statistics and Public Policy*, ed. Bruce D. Spencer (Oxford: Clarendon Press, 1997), 84–5.

40 Porter, *The Rise of Statistical Thinking*, 110.

41 Desrosières, *The Politics of Large Numbers*, 113.

42 Karl Pearson, *The Life, Letters and Labours of Francis Galton*, 3 vols (Cambridge: Cambridge University Press, 1924), 2:228.

43 Francis Galton, 'Composite Portraits', *Nature* 18, no. 447 (1878): 97–100; Francis Galton, 'Typical Laws of Heredity', *Nature* 15, no. 388–90 (1877): 492–5; 512–14; 532–3.

44 Galton, 'Composite Portraits', 97.

45 Gina Lombroso and Cesare Lombroso, *Criminal Man: According to the Classification of Cesare Lombroso* (New York: Putnam, 1911), 7.

46 Galton, 'Composite Portraits', 97–8.

47 Cryle and Stephens, *Normality: A Critical Genealogy*, 215–16.

48 R. Percy Smith, 'Sir George Henry Savage, MD, FRCP', *Journal of Mental Science* 67, no. 279 (1921): 402, 395.

49 Paul A. Lombardo, ed., *A Century of Eugenics in America: From the Indiana Experiment to the Human Genome Era* (Bloomington: Indiana University Press, 2010); Daniel J. Kevles, *In the Name of Eugenics: Genetics and the Uses of Human Heredity* (Cambridge, MA: Harvard University Press, 1995), 99.

50 For example, see Stephen Jay Gould, *The Mismeasure of Man* (Harmondsworth: Penguin, 1984), chap. 2.

51 Patrick Brantlinger, 'Victorians and Africans: The Genealogy of the Myth of the Dark Continent', *Critical Inquiry* 12, no. 1 (1985): 166–203.

52 William Booth, *In Darkest England, and the Way Out* (London and New York: Salvation Army, 1890), 9.

53 Booth, *In Darkest England*, 11.

54 Kevin R. Fontaine et al., 'Years of Life Lost Due to Obesity', *JAMA* 289, no. 2 (8 January 2003): 187–93.

55 I first heard about the hair gauge when one of my colleagues at UCL supervised a museum studies project investigating its heritage. For more on the results of this project, see www.ucl.ac.uk/culture/ucl-science-collections/eugen-fischers-hair-colour-gauge.

56 Anna Fazackerley, 'UCL Launches Inquiry into Historical Links With Eugenics', *Guardian*, 6 December 2018.

57 Bernard Rorke and Marek Szilvasi, 'Racism's Cruelest Cut: Coercive Sterilisation of Romani Women and Their Fight for Justice in the Czech Republic (1966–2016)', openDemocracy, accessed 2 August 2021, www.opendemocracy.net/en/can-europe-make-it/racisms-cruelest-cut-coercive-sterilization-of-roman/; Gwendolyn Albert and Marek Szilvasi, 'Intersectional Discrimination of Romani Women Forcibly Sterilized in the Former Czechoslovakia and Czech Republic', *Health and Human Rights Journal* 19, no. 2 (4 December 2017): 23–34.

2 Do I Have a Normal Body?

1 'British feet are "getting bigger and wider"', BBC News, 3 June 2014.

2 Size 5 to 11 in the US. The average US shoe size purchased in 1998 was 8.076 (UK size 5.5), with a standard deviation of 1.468.

3   Paul Valéry, 'Aesthetics', in *Collected Works in English*, vol. 13 (Princeton: Princeton University Press, 1964).

4   Shigehisa Kuriyama, *The Expressiveness of the Body and the Divergence of Greek and Chinese Medicine* (New York: Zone Books, 1999), 131.

5   Peter Cryle and Elizabeth Stephens, *Normality: A Critical Genealogy* (Chicago and London: University of Chicago Press, 2017), 296.

6   Anna G. Creadick, *Perfectly Average: The Pursuit of Normality in Postwar America* (Amherst and Boston: University of Massachusetts Press, 2010), 20–21.

7   Creadick, *Perfectly Average*, 28–36.

8   Alan Petersen, *The Body in Question: A Socio-Cultural Approach* (Abingdon: Routledge, 2007), 65; Sarah Grogan, *Body Image: Understanding Body Dissatisfaction in Men, Women and Children*, 2nd edn (London and New York: Routledge, 2008), 3.

9   Karl Pearson, *The Life, Letters and Labours of Francis Galton*, 3 vols (Cambridge: Cambridge University Press, 1924), 2:458.

10 Pearson, *Life of Galton*, 2:341.

11 Charles Darwin, *The Descent of Man, and Selection in Relation to Sex*, vol. 2 (London: John Murray, 1871), 355.

12 Darwin, *Descent of Man*, 2:350.

13 William Winwood Reade, *The Martyrdom of Man*, 11th edn (London: Trubner & Co., 1886), 455.

14 Reade, *Martyrdom of Man*, 455.

15 Sander L. Gilman, *Making the Body Beautiful: A Cultural History of Aesthetic Surgery* (Princeton: Princeton University Press, 1999), 85–7.

16 Petrus Camper, *The Works of the Late Professor Camper, on the Connexion between the Science of Anatomy, and the Art of Drawing, Painting, Statuary, &c., &c*, trans. T. Cogan (London: C. Dilly, 1794), 99.

17 Samuel Roberts Wells, *New Physiognomy* (New York: Fowler and Wells, 1867), 535–8.

18 Frances Eliza Kingsley, *Charles Kingsley: His Letters and Memories of His Life* (London and New York: Macmillan, 1899), 236.

19 Shoma Munshi, 'A Perfect 10 – "Modern and Indian": Representations of the Body in Beauty Pageants and the Visual Media in Contemporary India', in *Confronting the Body: The Politics of Physicality in Colonial and Post-Colonial India*, ed. James H. Mills and Satadru Sen (London: Anthem Press, 2004), 162.

20 Munshi, 'A Perfect 10', 162.

21 Petersen, *The Body in Question*, 76.

22 Remi Joseph-Salisbury, 'Afro Hair: How Pupils Are Tackling Discriminatory Uniform Policies', *The Conversation*, 20 April 2021.

23 Adolphe Quetelet, *A Treatise on Man and the Development of His Faculties*, trans. Robert Knox (Edinburgh: W. & R. Chambers, 1842), 64–6.

24 Ancel Keys et al., 'Indices of Relative Weight and Obesity', *Journal of Chronic Diseases* 25 (1972): 329–43.

25 Amy Erdman Farrell, *Fat Shame: Stigma and the Fat Body in American Culture* (New York and London: New York University Press, 2011), 34.

26 Farrell, *Fat Shame*, 27.

27 Silas Weir Mitchell, *Fat and Blood and How to Make Them*, 2nd edn (Philadelphia: J. B. Lippincott & Co., 1882), 25.

28 William Banting, *Letter on Corpulence, Addressed to the Public*, 5th edn (New York: Mohun, Ebbs & Hough, 1865), 6.

29 Farrell, *Fat Shame*, 38.

30 *Life Magazine*, 3 December 1914, 1042.

31 William Howard Hay, *Weight Control* (London: George G. Harrap, 1936), 21.

32 'Are our women scrawny?' *Harper's Bazaar*, 7 November 1896, 924.

33 Julien-Joseph Virey, *Natural History of the Negro Race*, ed. and trans. J. H. Guenebault (Charleston, SC: D. J. Dowling, 1837), 25.

34 Sabrina Strings, *Fearing the Black Body: The Racial Origins of Fat Phobia* (New York: New York University Press, 2019), 85–98.

35 Strings, *Fearing the Black Body*, 164.

36 Carl C. Seltzer, 'Limitations of Height–Weight Standards (Letters to the Editor)', *The New England Journal of Medicine* 272 (1965): 1132.

37 *Build and Blood Pressure Study* (Chicago: Society of Actuaries, 1959), 1.

38 Strings, *Fearing the Black Body*, 198.

39 Strings, *Fearing the Black Body*, 202.

40 Kevin R. Fontaine et al., 'Years of Life Lost Due to Obesity', *JAMA* 289, no. 2 (8 January 2003): 187–93.

41 Zuzanna Shonfield, *The Precariously Privileged: A Medical Man's Family in Victorian London* (Oxford: Oxford University Press, 1987).

42 *The Diary of Virginia Woolf*, ed. Anne Olivier Bell (New York: Harcourt, Brace, Jovanovich, 1980), 152.

43 George Croghan, *Army Life on the Western Frontier: Selections from the Official Reports Made Between 1826 and 1845*, ed. Francis Paul Prucha (Norman: University of Oklahoma Press, 2014), 59.

44 Robert Ross, *Clothing: A Global History* (Cambridge and Malden: Polity Press, 2008), 56–7.

45 Quoted in Stanley Chapman, 'The Innovating Entrepreneurs in the British Ready-Made Clothing Industry', *Textile History* 24, no. 1 (1993): 14–16.

46 Ross, *Clothing*, 121.

47 Ross, *Clothing*, 109, 114.

48 Mass Observation Archive: File Report no. 2045 'Women's Clothes in Chester', March 1944. Of course, wartime rationing undoubtedly had an impact on the proportion of clothes that were home-made or altered at this time.

49 Cryle and Stephens, *Normality: A Critical Genealogy*, 314.

50 Ruth O'Brien et al., *Women's Measurements for Garment and Pattern Construction* (Washington, DC: US Dept of Agriculture, 1941), 47.

51 'Freaks in Revolt', *Daily News*, 7 January 1899.

52 'The Revolt of the Freaks', *Standard*, 16 January 1899, 2.

53 Rosemarie Garland-Thomson, *Extraordinary Bodies: Figuring Physical Disability in American Culture and Literature* (New York: Columbia University Press, 1997), 61.

54 Rachel Adams, *Sideshow USA: Freaks and the American Cultural Imagination* (Chicago: University of Chicago Press, 2001), chap. 2; Garland-Thomson, *Extraordinary Bodies*, 62–3.

55 Arthur Goddard, '"Even as You and I": At Home with the Barnum Freaks', *English Illustrated Magazine*, no. 173 (February 1898), 495.

56 Adams, *Sideshow USA*, 30.

57 Nadja Durbach, *Spectacle of Deformity: Freak Shows and Modern British Culture* (Berkeley and Los Angeles: University of California Press, 2009), 92–3.

58 Adams, *Sideshow USA*, 40.

59 Tod Browning, *Freaks* (1932; 1947 reissue), dist. Dwain Esper.

60 Susan M. Schweik, *The Ugly Laws: Disability in Public* (New York: New York University Press, 2009).

61 Schweik, *Ugly Laws*, 6.

62 Schweik, *Ugly Laws*, 4–5.

63 Oliver Wendell Holmes, 'The Human Wheel, Its Spokes and Felloes', *Atlantic Monthly*, 1 May 1863, 574.

64 Schweik, *Ugly Laws*, 1.

65 Schweik, *Ugly Laws*, 3.

66 Lucy Wright and Amy M. Hamburger, *Education and Occupations of Cripples, Juvenile and Adult: A Survey of All the Cripples of Cleveland, Ohio, in 1916* (New York: Red Cross Institute for Crippled and Disabled Men, 1918), 222–3.

67 Holmes, 'The Human Wheel, Its Spokes and Felloes', 574.

68 Frances Bernstein, 'Prosthetic Manhood in the Soviet Union at the End of World War II', *Osiris* 30, no. 1 (18 January 2015): 113–33; Katherine Ott, 'Introduction', in *Artificial Parts, Practical Lives: Modern Histories of Prosthetics*, ed. Katherine Ott, David Serlin, and Stephen Mihm (New York: New York University Press, 2002).

69 Wright and Hamburger, *Education and Occupations*, 19.

70 Joanna Bourke, *Dismembering the Male: Men's Bodies, Britain and the Great War* (London: Reaktion, 1996), 44.

71 Office for National Statistics, *Updated estimates of coronavirus (COVID-19) related deaths by disability status January to 20 November 2020* (London: Office for National Statistics, 2021).

72 Daniel J. Wilson, 'Passing in the Shadow of FDR: Polio Survivors, Passing, and the Negotiation of Disability', in *Disability and Passing: Blurring the Lines of Identity*, ed. Jeffrey A. Brune and Daniel J. Wilson (Philadelphia: Temple University Press, 2013), 15.

73 The story was uncovered by Hugh Gallagher, himself a polio survivor. Hugh Gregory Gallagher, *FDR's Splendid Deception*, rev. edn (Arlington, VA: Vandamere Press, 1994).

74 Wilson, 'Passing in the Shadow of FDR'.

75 Wilson, 'Passing in the Shadow of FDR', 28.

76   George Bernard Shaw, *Plays: Pleasant and Unpleasant* (New York: Brentano's, 1906), vii.
77   More recent estimates put the proportion of people needing glasses or contact lenses at slightly lower, around three-quarters of the population. *Britain's Eye Health in Focus: A Snapshot of Consumer Attitudes and Behaviour towards Eye Health* (London: College of Optometrists, 2013).
78   Todd Rose, *The End of Average* (London: Penguin, 2015), 4.

3 Do I Have a Normal Mind?

1   D. L. Rosenhan, 'On Being Sane in Insane Places', *Science* 179, no. 4070 (19 January 1973): 379.
2   Robert L. Spitzer, 'On Pseudoscience in Science, Logic in Remission, and Psychiatric Diagnosis: A Critique of Rosenhan's "On Being Sane in Insane Places"', *Journal of Abnormal Psychology* 84, no. 5 (1975): 442–52; Susannah Cahalan, *The Great Pretender* (London: Canongate, 2020).
3   Rosenhan, 'On Being Sane in Insane Places', 380.
4   Nathan Filer, *The Heartland: Finding and Losing Schizophrenia* (London: Faber and Faber, 2019), 17.
5   Robert L. Spitzer et al., 'Schizophrenia and other psychotic disorders in DSM-III', *Schizophrenia Bulletin* 4 (1978): 493. See also DSM-III Task Force, *DSM-III: Diagnostic and Statistical Manual of Mental Disorders* (Washington, DC: American Psychiatric Association, 1980).
6   Henry Sidgwick et al., 'Report on the Census of Hallucinations', *Proceedings of the Society for Psychical Research* 10 (1894): 73–4.
7   See Christopher Chabris and Daniel Simons's 2010 video at www. theinvisiblegorilla.com/gorilla_experiment.html.
8   Mary Boyle, *Schizophrenia: A Scientific Delusion?* (London: Routledge, 1990).
9   Michael MacDonald, *Mystical Bedlam: Madness, Anxiety, and Healing in Seventeenth-Century England* (Cambridge: Cambridge University Press, 1981), 200.
10   Daniel Hack Tuke, *Illustrations of the Influence of the Mind upon the Body in Health and Disease*, vol. 1, 2nd edn (London: J. & A. Churchill, 1884), viii.
11   Edmund Gurney, Frederic William Henry Myers, and Frank Podmore, *Phantasms of the Living* (London: Trubner and Co., 1886), x.
12   Sidgwick et al., 'Report on the Census of Hallucinations'. See also Christopher Keep, 'Evidence in Matters Extraordinary: Numbers, Narratives, and the Census of Hallucinations', *Victorian Studies* 61, no. 4 (2019): 582–607; Andreas Sommer, 'Professional Heresy: Edmund Gurney (1847–1888) and the Study of Hallucinations and Hypnotism', *Medical History* 55 (2014): 383–8.
13   Gurney, Myers, and Podmore, *Phantasms of the Living*, 499.
14   Boyle, *Schizophrenia*, 198.

15 For a detailed and personal account of the network, see Gail A. Hornstein, *Agnes's Jacket: A Psychologist's Search for the Meanings of Madness* (New York: Rodale, 2009).

16 'HVN: A Positive Approach to Voices and Visions', accessed 12 January 2022, www.hearing-voices.org/about-us/hvn-values.

17 Theo B. Hyslop, *The Borderland: Some of the Problems of Insanity* (London: Philip Allan & Co., 1925), 1–2.

18 For a brief overview of Hyslop's life, see W. H. B. Stoddart, 'Obituary: T. B. Hyslop', *British Medical Journal* 1, no. 3764 (1933): 347. No one else has written much about him.

19 See John MacGregor, *The Discovery of the Art of the Insane* (Princeton: Princeton University Press, 1992), 162–3.

20 Anonymous [Theo B. Hyslop], *Laputa, Revisited by Gulliver Redivivus in 1905*, 2nd edn (London: Hirschfeld, 1905), 39.

21 Theo B. Hyslop, *The Great Abnormals* (London: Philip Allan & Co., 1925), v.

22 Hyslop, *Great Abnormals*, 275.

23 Theo B. Hyslop, *Mental Physiology: Especially in Its Relations to Mental Disorders* (London: J. & A. Churchill, 1895), 469.

24 Andrew Wynter, *The Borderlands of Insanity* (London: Renshaw, 1877), 42.

25 George Savage, 'An Address on the Borderland of Insanity', *British Medical Journal* 1, no. 2357 (1906): 489–92.

26 The Victorians were very worried about wrongful confinement in asylums, which is one reason why so many Victorian novels hinge on wrongful diagnosis – not, as modern readers often assume, because cases like the Lanchester one were common at the time. 'The Lanchester Case, of Insanity and the New "Morality"', *The Lancet* 146, no. 3767 (1895): 1175–6.

27 'The Lanchester Case', *Journal of Mental Science* 42 (1896): 134–6.

28 Kieran McNally, *A Critical History of Schizophrenia* (Basingstoke and New York: Palgrave Macmillan, 2016), 199.

29 Samuel A. Cartwright, 'Report on the Diseases and Physical Peculiarities of the Negro Race', *The New Orleans Medical And Surgical Journal* (1851), 708.

30 Cartwright, 'Report on the Diseases', 708.

31 Silas Weir Mitchell, *Fat and Blood and How to Make Them*, 2nd edn (Philadelphia: J. B. Lippincott & Co., 1882).

32 Elaine Showalter, *The Female Malady: Women, Madness and English Culture, 1830–1980* (London: Virago, 1987).

33 George Miller Beard, *A Practical Treatise on Nervous Exhaustion (Neurasthenia)* (New York: E. B. Treat, 1889), 1.

34 Female Patient Casebook for 1895 (CB 152), Bethlem Museum of the Mind, entry 79.

35 Voluntary Boarders Casebook, 1893–5 (CB 147), Bethlem Museum of the Mind, entry 66.

36 George Savage, 'Marriage in Neurotic Subjects', *Journal of Mental Science* 29 (1883): 49.

37 Wynter, *Borderlands of Insanity*, 57.

38 Hyslop, *Mental Physiology*, 469.

39 Rocco J. Gennaro, 'Psychopathologies and Theories of Consciousness: An Overview', in *Disturbed Consciousness: New Essays on Psychopathology and Theories of Consciousness* (Cambridge, MA and London: MIT Press, 2015), 3.

40 Theo B. Hyslop, 'On "Double Consciousness"', *British Medical Journal* 2, no. 2021 (1899): 782–6.

41 Ian Hacking, *Rewriting the Soul: Multiple Personality and the Sciences of Memory* (Princeton: Princeton University Press, 1998), 166–7.

42 Pierre Janet, *L'automatisme psychologique: Essai de psychologie expérimentale sur les formes inférieures de l'activité humaine* (Paris: Félix Alcan, 1889), 89.

43 Sigmund Freud and Josef Breuer, *Studies on Hysteria*, ed. Angela Richards and James Strachey, trans. James Strachey, rev. edn (Harmondsworth: Penguin, 1991), 74.

44 Freud and Breuer, *Studies on Hysteria*, 77.

45 Freud and Breuer, *Studies on Hysteria*, 95.

46 Mikkel Borch-Jacobsen, 'Making Psychiatric History: Madness as Folie à Plusieurs', *History of the Human Sciences* 14, no. 2 (2001): 29.

47 See Sonu Shamdasani, 'Psychotherapy: The Invention of a Word', *History of the Human Sciences* 18, no. 1 (2005): 1–22; Tuke, *Illustrations*, 2:231–85.

48 Letter from Freud to Carl Jung, 3 January 1913. *The Freud/Jung Letters: The Correspondence between Sigmund Freud and C. G. Jung*, ed. William McGuire, trans. Ralph Manheim and R. F. C. Hull (Princeton: Princeton University Press, 1974), 539.

49 *Mental Health: New Understanding, New Hope* (Geneva: WHO, 2001), 23.

50 Stephen Ginn and Jamie Horder, '"One in Four" with a Mental Health Problem: The Anatomy of a Statistic', *BMJ* 344 (22 February 2012).

51 Ginn and Horder, '"One in Four"', 2.

52 Jamie Horder, 'How True Is the One-in-Four Mental Health Statistic?' *Guardian*, 24 April 2010.

53 Paul C. Horton, 'Normality: Toward a Meaningful Construct', *Comprehensive Psychiatry* 12, no. 1 (1971): 57–9.

54 Alfred H. Stanton and Morris S. Schwartz, *The Mental Hospital: A Study of Institutional Participation in Psychiatric Illness and Treatment* (New York: Basic Books, 1954), 144.

55 Kwame McKenzie and Kamaldeep Bhui, 'Institutional Racism in Mental Health Care', *BMJ* 334, no. 7595 (31 March 2007): 649–50.

56 Care Quality Commission, 'Count Me in 2010: Results of the 2010 national census of inpatients and patients on supervised community treatment in mental health and learning disability services in England and Wales' (April 2011), www.mentalhealthlaw.co.uk/media/CQC_Count_me_in_2010.pdf.

4 Is My Sex Life Normal?

1   Liz Stanley, *Sex Surveyed 1949–1994: From Mass-Observation's "Little Kinsey" to the National Survey and the Hite Reports* (London: Taylor and Francis, 1995), 166.

2   Samuel-Auguste Tissot, *Diseases Caused by Masturbation* (Philadelphia and New York: Gottfried & Fritz, 2015), 19–20.

3   Thomas Laqueur, *Solitary Sex: A Cultural History of Masturbation* (New York: Zone Books, 2003).

4   *Onania: or, the Heinous Sin of Self-Pollution, and All Its Frightful Consequences (in Both Sexes), Considered* (London: P. Varenne bookseller, 1716).

5   *Onania*, 99–101.

6   Laqueur, *Solitary Sex*, 17–19.

7   Robert Ritchie, 'An Inquiry into a Frequent Cause of Insanity in Young Men', *The Lancet* 77, no. 1955–60 (1861): 159.

8   James Paget, *Clinical Lectures and Essays*, ed. Howard Marsh (London: Longmans, Green and Co., 1879), 292.

9   David Yellowlees, 'Masturbation', in *Dictionary of Psychological Medicine*, ed. Daniel Hack Tuke, vol. 2 (London: J. & A. Churchill, 1892), 784.

10 Clement Dukes, *The Preservation of Health as It Is Affected by Personal Habits: Such as Cleanliness, Temperance, etc.* (London: Rivington, 1884).

11 Havelock Ellis, *Studies in the Psychology of Sex: The Evolution of Modesty; the Phenomena of Sexual Periodicity; Auto-erotism* (Philadelphia: F. A. Davis Company, 1901), 115.

12 Ellis, *Studies: The Evolution of Modesty*, 118.

13 George J. Makari, 'Between Seduction and Libido: Sigmund Freud's Masturbation Hypotheses and the Realignment of His Etiologic Thinking, 1897–1905', *Bulletin of the History of Medicine* 72, no. 4 (1998): 655–6.

14 'Contributions to a Discussion on Masturbation' (1912), in *The Standard Edition of the Complete Psychological Works of Sigmund Freud*, ed. and trans. James Strachey, vol. 12 (London: Hogarth Press, 1958), 239–54.

15 Lesley A. Hall, 'Forbidden by God, Despised by Men: Masturbation, Medical Warnings, Moral Panic, and Manhood in Great Britain, 1850–1950', *Journal of the History of Sexuality* 2, no. 3 (1992): 386.

16 Quoted in Hall, 'Forbidden by God', 383–4. See letter dated 24 September 1927 (Wellcome Library PP/MCS/A.189).

17 Stanley, *Sex Surveyed*, 79–81.

18 Letter from Marie Stopes, typed postscript dated 27 September 1927 (Wellcome Library PP/MCS/A.189).

19 Eustace Chesser, *Grow Up – And Live* (Harmondsworth: Penguin, 1949), 243.

20 Katharine Angel, 'The History of "Female Sexual Dysfunction" as a Mental Disorder in the Twentieth Century', *Current Opinion in Psychiatry*, 23:6 (2010), 537.

21 Mass Observation Archive, MOA12, 12-12-A, img. 9426.

22 Hall, 'Forbidden by God', 386; Marjorie Proops, *Dear Marje ...* (London: Andre Deutsch, 1976), 60.

23 Neil McKenna, *Fanny and Stella: The Young Men Who Shocked Victorian England* (London: Faber and Faber, 2013), 6.

24 Cited in Michelle Liu Carriger, '"The Unnatural History and Petticoat Mystery of Boulton and Park": A Victorian Sex Scandal and the Theatre Defense', *TDR: The Drama Review* 57, no. 4 (2013): 135.

25 'Police', *The Times*, 30 April 1870, 11.

26 Charles Upchurch, 'Forgetting the Unthinkable: Cross-Dressers and British Society in the Case of the Queen vs Boulton and Others', *Gender & History* 12, no. 1 (2000): 137.

27 McKenna, *Fanny and Stella*, 35.

28 Judith Rowbotham, 'A Deception on the Public: The Real Scandal of Boulton and Park', *Liverpool Law Review* 36 (2015): 126.

29 Rowbotham, 'A Deception on the Public', 127; 130.

30 For additional examples of medical writers who used 'normal' and 'abnormal' relationally when talking about sex, see Peter Cryle and Elizabeth Stephens, *Normality: A Critical Genealogy* (Chicago and London: University of Chicago Press, 2017), 288.

31 Matt Cook, '"A New City of Friends": London and Homosexuality in the 1890s', *History Workshop Journal* 56 (2003): 36.

32 Jack Saul, *Sins of the Cities of the Plain* (Paris: Olympia Press, 2006).

33 Cook, '"A New City of Friends"', 40.

34 Cook, '"A New City of Friends"', 51–2.

35 Criminal Law Amendment Act, 1885, 48 & 49 Vict. c 69, section 11. In 1871, similar laws were adopted across Germany following unification, copying existing laws in Austria.

36 R. von Krafft-Ebing, *Psychopathia Sexualis, with Especial Reference to the Antipathic Sexual Instinct: A Medico-Forensic Study*, trans. F. J. Rebman, 2nd English edn (New York: Medical Art Agency, 1906), 196–7.

37 Krafft-Ebing, *Psychopathia Sexualis*, viii.

38 Renate Irene Hauser, 'Sexuality, Neurasthenia and the Law: Richard von Krafft-Ebing (1840–1902)' (PhD diss., UCL, 1992).

39 Krafft-Ebing, *Psychopathia Sexualis*, 294.

40 Krafft-Ebing, *Psychopathia Sexualis*, 382.

41 Catharine Cox Miles and Lewis M. Terman, *Sex and Personality: Studies in Masculinity and Femininity* (New York and London: McGraw Hill, 1936), 6.

42 Miles and Terman, *Sex and Personality*, 9.

43 Michael C. C. Adams, *The Best War Ever: America and World War II* (Baltimore: Johns Hopkins University Press, 1994), 78.

44 Samuel A. Stouffer, ed., *The American Soldier: Combat and Its Aftermath*, vol. 2, Studies in Social Psychology in World War II (Princeton: Princeton University Press, 1949), 523.

45 Anna G. Creadick, *Perfectly Average: The Pursuit of Normality in Postwar America* (Amherst and Boston: University of Massachusetts Press, 2010), 92.

46 Katie Sutton, 'Kinsey and the Psychoanalysts: Cross-Disciplinary Knowledge Production in Post-War US Sex Research', *History of the Human Sciences* 34, no. 1 (2021): 132.

47 Creadick, *Perfectly Average*, 93.

48 Tommy Dickinson et al., '"Queer" Treatments: Giving a Voice to Former Patients Who Received Treatments for Their "Sexual Deviations"', *Journal of Clinical Nursing* 21, no. 9–10 (2012): 1346.

49 Havelock Ellis, *My Life* (London and Toronto: William Heinemann, 1940), 250–51.

50 Ellis, *My Life*, 254.

51 Ellis, *My Life*, 263. Although, Ellis was actually already in touch with John Addington Symonds at this time, and discussing the topic in letters, so his memoirs are perhaps not entirely accurate on the order of events.

52 Ellis, *My Life*, 264.

53 Ellis, *My Life*, 179.

54 Ellis, *Studies: The Evolution of Modesty*, vi.

55 Ellis, *My Life*, 263.

56 Havelock Ellis and John Addington Symonds, *Sexual Inversion: A Critical Edition*, ed. Ivan Crozier (Basingstoke: Palgrave Macmillan, 2008), 34–5. This was the first volume of Ellis's studies to be published (it later became volume 2 of the series), written in collaboration with gay poet and essayist John Addington Symonds.

57 Havelock Ellis and John Addington Symonds, *Studies in the Psychology of Sex: Sexual Inversion* (London: Wilson & MacMillan, 1897), 94.

58 Patricia Cotti, 'Freud and the Sexual Drive before 1905: From Hesitation to Adoption', *History of the Human Sciences* 21, no. 3 (2008): 37.

59 Paul H. Gebhard and Alan B. Johnson, *The Kinsey Data: Marginal Tabulations of the 1938–1963 Interviews Conducted by the Institute for Sex Research* (Philadelphia: W. B. Saunders Company, 1979), 2.

60 Donna J. Drucker, *The Classification of Sex: Alfred Kinsey and the Organization of Knowledge* (Pittsburgh: University of Pittsburgh Press, 2014), 119.

61 Gebhard and Johnson, *The Kinsey Data*, 19.

62 Alfred C. Kinsey, Wardell B. Pomeroy, and Clyde E. Martin, *Sexual Behavior in the Human Male* (Philadelphia and London: W. B. Saunders Company, 1949), 637–9.

63 Kinsey, Pomeroy, and Martin, *Sexual Behavior*, 610.

64 Kinsey, Pomeroy, and Martin, *Sexual Behavior*, 666.

65 Drucker, *Classification of Sex*, 77.

66 Drucker, *Classification of Sex*, 118.

67 All these completed surveys can be found in Mass Observation Archive 12, folders 12-2-C; 12-9-G; 12-12-A to 12-12-E; and 12-13-A to 12-13-F.

68 Stanley, *Sex Surveyed*, 199.

69 One respondent did not explicitly identify as the gender they were born as.

70 Mass Observation Archive: 12-13-D, img. 10734.

71 Bob Erens et al., 'National Survey of Sexual Attitudes and Lifestyles II: Reference Tables and Summary', 2003, 8.

72 Stanley, *Sex Surveyed*, 51.

73 Tim Cornwell, 'George Michael Arrested Over "Lewd Act"', *Independent*, 9 April 1998.

74 Krafft-Ebing, *Psychopathia Sexualis*, 381.

75 John Gray, *Men Are from Mars, Women Are from Venus* (New York: HarperCollins, 1992).

76 Laura Gowing, *Common Bodies: Women, Touch and Power in Seventeenth-Century England* (New Haven and London: Yale University Press, 2003).

77 Thomas Laqueur, *Making Sex: Body and Gender from the Greeks to Freud* (Cambridge, MA and London: Harvard University Press, 1990).

78 Laqueur, *Making Sex*; Carol Groneman, 'Nymphomania: The Historical Construction of Female Sexuality', *Signs* 19, no. 2 (1994): 345–6.

79 Groneman, 'Nymphomania', 350; Ivan Crozier, 'William Acton and the History of Sexuality: The Medical and Professional Context', *Journal of Victorian Culture* 5, no. 1 (2000): 12.

80 William Acton, *The Functions and Disorders of the Reproductive Organs*, 4th edn (London: John Churchill, 1865), 112.

81 Terri D. Fisher, Zachary T. Moore, and Mary-Jo Pittenger, 'Sex on the Brain?: An Examination of Frequency of Sexual Cognitions as a Function of Gender, Erotophilia, and Social Desirability', *Journal of Sex Research* 49, no. 1 (1 January 2012): 69–77.

82 Groneman, 'Nymphomania', 341.

83 Groneman, 'Nymphomania', 337–8.

84 Groneman, 'Nymphomania', 352.

85 Ornella Moscucci, 'Clitoridectomy, Circumcision, and the Politics of Sexual Pleasure in Mid-Victorian Britain', in *Sexualities in Victorian Britain*, ed. Andrew H. Miller and James Eli Adams (Bloomington: Indiana University Press, 1996), 61.

86 Moscucci, 'Clitoridectomy', 68.

87 Andrew T. Scull, '"A Chance to Cut Is a Chance to Cure": Sexual Surgery for Psychosis in Three Nineteenth-Century Societies', in *Psychiatry and Social Control in the Nineteenth and Twentieth Centuries* (London and New York: Routledge, 2006), 160.

88 Female Patient Casebook for 1888 (CB 135), Bethlem Museum of the Mind, entry 148.

89 Josephine Butler, *Recollections of George Butler* (Bristol: Arrowsmith, 1896), 183.

90 Judith R. Walkowitz, *City of Dreadful Delight: Narratives of Sexual Danger in Late-Victorian London* (London: Virago, 1992), 88–9.

91 Butler, *Recollections of George Butler*, 194.

92 Ruth Hall, *Dear Dr Stopes: Sex in the 1920s* (London: Andre Deutsch, 1978), 162.

93 Drucker, *Classification of Sex*, 163.

94 From Lawrence's unpublished autobiography, quoted in Sutton, 'Kinsey and the Psychoanalysts', 139.

95 Sutton, 'Kinsey and the Psychoanalysts', 139.

96 Hera Cook, *The Long Sexual Revolution: English Women, Sex, and Contraception 1800–1975* (Oxford: Oxford University Press, 2005), 179.

97 Stanley, *Sex Surveyed*, 139.

98 Stanley, *Sex Surveyed*, 139.

99 Mass Observation Archive: 12-9-G / A-9-4, img. 7365.

100 Cook, *Long Sexual Revolution*, 289.

101 Susanna Kaysen, *Girl, Interrupted* (New York: Random House, 1993), 11.

102 Kaysen, *Girl, Interrupted*, 158.

103 Diane Francis, 'Sex, Cancer and the Perils of Promiscuity', *Maclean's*, 6 October 1980.

104 Sabrina Strings, *Fearing the Black Body: The Racial Origins of Fat Phobia* (New York: New York University Press, 2019), 81–2.

105 Sue Jackson, '"I'm 15 and Desperate for Sex": "Doing" and "Undoing" Desire in Letters to a Teenage Magazine', *Feminism & Psychology* 15, no. 3 (2005): 301; 304.

106 Jackson, '"I'm 15"', 305–6.

107 Samuel Osborne, 'Study Suggests "Ideal Number of Sexual Partners" to Have', *Independent*, 21 January 2016.

108 Claire R. Gravelin, Monica Biernat, and Caroline E. Bucher, 'Blaming the Victim of Acquaintance Rape: Individual, Situational, and Sociocultural Factors', *Frontiers in Psychology* 9 (2019): 2422. See also Joanna Bourke, *Rape: A History from 1860 to the Present* (London: Virago, 2007).

109 Michael Warner, 'Introduction: Fear of a Queer Planet', *Social Text* 29 (1991): 6.

110 For a fascinating analysis of the variety of ways the term is used in gender and sexuality studies, see Joseph Marchia and Jamie M. Sommer, '(Re) Defining Heteronormativity', *Sexualities* 22, no. 3 (2019): 267–95.

111 Mass Observation Archive, 'Sexual Behaviour 1939–1950', Topic Collection 12, Box 12, A9-2, 12-12-E, img. 9836.

5 Is This a Normal Way to Feel?

1 William James, 'What Is an Emotion?', *Mind* 9, no. 34 (1884): 188–205.

2 Georges Dreyfus, 'Is Compassion an Emotion? A Cross-Cultural Exploration of Mental Typologies', in *Visions of Compassion: Western Scientists and Tibetan Buddhists Examine Human Nature*, ed. Richard J. Davidson and Anne Harrington (Oxford: Oxford University Press, 2002), 31–2.

3 Translation of Saint-Just's unfinished essay in William Reddy, *The Navigation of Feeling: A Framework for the History of Emotions* (Cambridge: Cambridge University Press, 2001), 177.

4 Thomas Dixon, *From Passions to Emotions: The Creation of a Secular Psychological Category* (Cambridge: Cambridge University Press, 2003), 98–134.

5 Entry for Tuesday, 26 March 1667, in *The Diary of Samuel Pepys*, ed. Henry B. Wheatley (London: George Bell and Sons, 1893).

6 Erin Sullivan, *Beyond Melancholy: Sadness and Selfhood in Renaissance England* (Oxford: Oxford University Press, 2016), 53.

7 Sullivan, *Beyond Melancholy*, 58.

8 Charles Féré, *The Pathology of Emotions: Physiological and Clinical Studies*, trans. Robert Park (London: University Press, 1899).

9 Daniel Hack Tuke, *Illustrations of the Influence of the Mind upon the Body in Health and Disease*, vol. 2, 2nd edn (London: J. & A. Churchill, 1884).

10 Peter Taggart et al., 'Anger, Emotion, and Arrhythmias: From Brain to Heart', *Frontiers in Physiology* 2 (2011): 67.

11 Johann Wolfgang von Goethe, *The Sorrows of Young Werther*, trans. Michael Hulse (London: Penguin Books, 1989), 23.

12 Michael MacDonald and Terence R. Murphy, *Sleepless Souls: Suicide in Early Modern England* (Oxford and New York: Oxford University Press, 1990), 190–92.

13 Charles S. Peirce, 'Evolutionary Love', *The Monist* 3, no. 2 (1893): 181.

14 Forbes Winslow, *The Anatomy of Suicide* (London: Henry Renshaw, 1840), 83.

15 Reddy, *Navigation of Feeling*, 216.

16 Thomas Dixon, 'The Tears of Mr Justice Willes', *Journal of Victorian Culture* 17, no. 1 (2012): 1–23.

17 J. A. Mangan, 'Social Darwinism and Upper-Class Education in Late Victorian and Edwardian England', in *Manliness and Morality: Middle-Class Masculinity in Britain and America, 1800–1940*, ed. J. A. Mangan and James Walvin (Manchester: Manchester University Press, 1995), 143.

18 Andrew Combe, *The Management of Infancy, Physiological and Moral*, revised and ed. James Clark, 10th edn (Edinburgh: Maclachlan and Stewart, 1870), 197.

19 H. Clay Trumbull, *Hints on Child-Training* (Philadelphia: J. D. Wattles, 1891), 95.

20 Thomas Dixon, *Weeping Britannia: Portrait of a Nation in Tears* (Oxford: Oxford University Press, 2015), 202.

21 Mass Observation Archive: Directive Replies, August 1950, participant 105.

22 William Moulton Marston, *Emotions of Normal People* (London: Kegan Paul, Trench, Trubner & Co., 1928), 1–2.

23 Both women had children with Marston, and continued to live together for decades after Marston's early death. For more on the family's unconventional life, see Jill Lepore, *The Secret History of Wonder Woman* (Melbourne: Scribe, 2015).

24 Marston, *Emotions of Normal People*, 394–6.

25 Lepore, *Secret History of Wonder Woman*, 180.

26 Karl A. Menninger, *Man Against Himself* (San Diego, New York and London: Harcourt, Brace, Jovanovich, 1985).

27 Frieda Fromm-Reichmann, *Principles of Intensive Psychotherapy* (Chicago: University of Chicago Press, 1950).

28   *Control Your Emotions I* (Buffalo, New York: Board of Education, 1950; n.p.:
      AV Geeks, 2020), avgeeks.com/control-your-emotions-1950.

29   Carol Zisowitz Stearns and Peter N. Stearns, *Anger: The Struggle for Emotional
      Control in America's History* (Chicago: University of Chicago Press, 1986), 4.

30   W. Lloyd Warner, *American Life: Dream and Reality* (Chicago: University of
      Chicago Press, 1962), 108–10.

31   Stearns and Stearns, *Anger*, 211.

32   Thomas Dixon, 'What Is the History of Anger a History Of?', *Emotions:
      History, Culture, Society* 4, no. 1 (14 September 2020): 6.

33   Ferdinand J. M. Lefebvre, *Louise Lateau of Bois d'Haine: Her Life, Her Ecstasies,
      and Her Stigmata: A Medical Study*, trans. Charles J. Bowen and E. MacKey,
      ed. James Spencer Northcote (London: Burns and Oates, 1873).

34   'Louise Lateau', *The Lancet* 97, no. 2486 (1871): 543–4.

35   Meredith Clymer, 'Ecstasy and Other Dramatic Disorders of the Nervous
      System', *Journal of Psychological Medicine* 4, no. 4 (1870): 658.

36   Pamela J. Walker, *Pulling the Devil's Kingdom Down: The Salvation Army in
      Victorian Britain* (Berkeley: University of California Press, 2001), 103–15.

37   Thomas F. G. Coates, *The Prophet of the Poor: The Life-Story of General Booth*
      (New York: E. P. Dutton and Co., 1906), 116.

38   'Rowdy Religion', *Saturday Review of Politics, Literature, Science and Art* 57, no.
      1492 (31 May 1884): 700.

39   'Lord Curzon's 15 Good Reasons Against the Grant of Female Suffrage'
      (pamphlet; NLS 1937.21(82), *c*.1910–14), digital.nls.uk/suffragettes/sources/
      source-24.html.

40   Edward Raymond Turner, 'The Women's Suffrage Movement in England',
      American Political Science Review 7, no. 4 (November 1913): 600.

41   Herbert Spencer, 'The Comparative Psychology of Man', *Mind* 1, no. 1
      (1876): 12.

42   William Winwood Reade, *Savage Africa: The Narrative of a Tour* (New York:
      Harper & Brothers, 1864), 426–7.

43   William Winwood Reade, *The African Sketch-Book*, vol. 2 (London: Smith,
      Elder & Co., 1873), 260.

44   J. D. Hargreaves, 'Winwood Reade and the Discovery of Africa', *African
      Affairs* 56, no. 225 (1957): 308.

45   William Winwood Reade, *The Martyrdom of Man*, 11th edn (London:
      Trubner & Co., 1886), 385.

46   British Association for the Advancement of Science, *Notes and Queries on
      Anthropology, for the Use of Travellers and Residents in Uncivilized Lands* (London:
      Edward Stanford, 1874), 13.

47   Spencer, 'The Comparative Psychology of Man', 8.

48   'Louise Lateau', *The Lancet* 104.2669 (1874): 604.

49   Almroth Edward Wright, *The Unexpurgated Case Against Woman Suffrage* (New
      York: Paul B. Hoeber, 1913), 165–88.

50   Ethel Smyth, 'Mrs Pankhurst's Treatment in Prison', *The Times*,
      19 April 1912.

51 Anna North, 'Attacks on Greta Thunberg Expose the Stigma Autistic Girls Face', *Vox*, 12 December 2019.

52 Joseph Henrich, *The Weirdest People in the World: How the West Became Psychologically Peculiar and Particularly Prosperous* (New York and London: Allen Lane, 2020), 50–52.

53 Edwin Balmer and William MacHarg, *The Achievements of Luther Trant* (Boston: Small, Maynard & Co., 1910), 38.

54 Balmer and MacHarg, *Achievements of Luther Trant*, foreword.

55 Balmer and MacHarg, *Achievements of Luther Trant*, 352.

56 William Davies, *The Happiness Industry: How the Government and Big Business Sold Us Well-Being* (London: Verso, 2015), 58.

57 W. Stanley Jevons, *The Theory of Political Economy* (London and New York: Macmillan, 1871), 13.

58 Francis Y. Edgeworth, *Mathematical Psychics* (London: C. Kegan Paul & Co., 1881), 101.

59 Charles Darwin, *The Expression of the Emotions in Man and Animals* (London: John Murray, 1872), 310.

60 Cesare Lombroso, *Criminal Man*, trans. Mary Gibson and Nicole Hahn Rafter (Durham, NC and London: Duke University Press, 2006), 210.

61 Geoffrey C. Bunn, *The Truth Machine: A Social History of the Lie Detector* (Baltimore: Johns Hopkins University Press, 2012), 146–7.

62 'Lie Detector Test Proves Bloodhounds Are Liars', *The New York Times*, 11 November 1935.

63 Charles F. Bond et al., 'Lie Detection across Cultures', *Journal of Nonverbal Behavior* 14, no. 3 (1 September 1990): 189–204.

64 Such as the Turkish lie detector developed in Istanbul in 2015. Belgin Akaltan and Ines Bensalem, 'Lie Detector Machine Designed Especially for Turks Being Developed', *Hurriyet Daily News*, 13 June 2015.

65 David T. Lykken, *A Tremor in the Blood: Uses and Abuses of the Lie Detector* (New York: Plenum Trade, 1998).

66 Daniel Hack Tuke, 'Case of Moral Insanity or Congenital Moral Defect, with Commentary', *Journal of Mental Science* 31, no. 135 (1885): 360–66.

67 Tuke, 'Case of Moral Insanity', 365.

68 Tuke, *Illustrations*, 2:285.

69 Tuke, 'Case of Moral Insanity', 363.

70 George Savage and Charles Arthur Mercier, 'Insanity of Conduct', *Journal of Mental Science* 42, no. 176 (1896), 1–17.

71 Albert Wilson, *Unfinished Man: A Scientific Analysis of the Psychopath or Human Degenerate* (London: Greening & Co., 1910), 3.

72 Wilson, *Unfinished Man*, 6.

73 Wilson, *Unfinished Man*, 3.

74 Wilson, *Unfinished Man*, 6.

75 Stephen Jay Gould, *The Mismeasure of Man* (Harmondsworth: Penguin, 1984), chap. 1.

76 Susanna Shapland, 'Defining the Elephant: A History of Psychopathy,
    1891–1959' (PhD diss., Birkbeck, University of London, 2019).
77 *Understanding Aggression* (London: Ministry of Health, 1960).
78 David Kennedy Henderson, 'Psychopathic States', *Journal of Mental Science*
    88, no. 373 (October 1942): 33.
79 David Kennedy Henderson, *Psychopathic States* (London: Chapman & Hall,
    1939), 129.
80 Hervey M. Cleckley, *The Mask of Sanity*, rev. edn (New York: New American
    Library, 1982), 212–13.
81 Robert D. Hare, *Without Conscience: The Disturbing World of the Psychopaths
    Among Us* (New York: Pocket Books, 1993), 44.
82 James Fallon, *The Psychopath Inside: A Neuroscientist's Personal Journey into the
    Dark Side of the Brain* (New York: Current, 2013), 112.
83 Jon Ronson, *The Psychopath Test: A Journey Through the Madness Industry*
    (London: Picador, 2011).
84 Philip K. Dick, *Do Androids Dream of Electric Sheep?* (London: Orion, 2011), 2.
85 Carlos Crivelli et al., 'The Fear Gasping Face as a Threat Display in a
    Melanesian Society', *Proceedings of the National Academy of Sciences* 113, no. 44
    (1 November 2016): 12403–7.
86 Tuan Le Mau et al., 'Professional Actors Demonstrate Variability,
    Not Stereotypical Expressions, When Portraying Emotional States in
    Photographs', *Nature Communications* 12, no. 1 (19 August 2021): 5037.

6 Are My Kids Normal?

1   Philip Larkin, 'This Be the Verse', in *High Windows* (London and Boston:
    Faber and Faber, 1986), 30.
2   Nancy Shute, 'To Succeed at Breast-Feeding, Most New Moms Could Use
    Help', *NPR*, 23 September 2013.
3   Katharina Rowold, 'Modern Mothers, Modern Babies: Breastfeeding and
    Mother's Milk in Interwar Britain', *Women's History Review* 28, no. 7 (2019):
    1163.
4   Anna Davin, 'Imperialism and Motherhood', *History Workshop Journal* 5
    (1978): 10.
5   George Newman, *Infant Mortality: A Social Problem* (New York: E. P. Dutton
    and Co., 1907), vi.
6   Newman, *Infant Mortality*, 221.
7   Maud Pember Reeves, *Round About a Pound a Week* (London: Persephone
    Books, 2008), 90–91; Newman, *Infant Mortality*, 249.
8   George Rosen, *A History of Public Health*, rev. edn (Baltimore: Johns Hopkins
    University Press, 2015), 205.
9   Davin, 'Imperialism and Motherhood', 11.
10 Greta Allen, *Practical Hints to Health Visitors* (London: The Scientific Press,
    1905), 5–6.

11   L. Emmett Holt, *The Diseases of Infancy and Childhood, for the Use of Students and Practitioners of Medicine* (New York: D. Appleton and Company, 1902), 18–21.

12   Enid Eve, *Manual for Health Visitors and Infant Welfare Workers* (New York: Wood, 1921), 80.

13   Davin, 'Imperialism and Motherhood', 41.

14   Rowold, 'Modern Mothers', 1168.

15   Eve, *Manual for Health Visitors*, 35.

16   Eve, *Manual for Health Visitors*, 33.

17   London County Council and W. H. Hamer, *Annual Report of the Council, 1914*, vol. 3, *Public Health* (London: London County Council, 1915), 96–7.

18   Reeves, *Round About a Pound*, 23–4.

19   Reeves, *Round About a Pound*, 169.

20   Reeves, *Round About a Pound*, 174–8.

21   Reeves, *Round About a Pound*, 84–5.

22   B. C. Stevens, *Annual Report on the Health, Sanitary Conditions, etc. of the Urban District of Barnes* (London: Urban District Council of Barnes, 1918), 21; Rowold, 'Modern Mothers', 1163.

23   'Vitamines', *The Times*, 25 November 1919.

24   Walthamstow Urban District Council, *Report of the Medical Officer of Health and School Medical Officer for the Year 1925* (London, 1925), 90.

25   Mila I. Pierce, 'A Nutritional Survey of School Children in Oxfordshire, London, and Birmingham', *Proceedings of the Royal Society of Medicine* 37, no. 7 (1944): 313–16.

26   Ronald S. Illingworth, *The Normal Child* (London: J. & A. Churchill, 1953), 85.

27   Ministry of Health, *Standards of Normal Weight in Infancy* (London: HMSO, 1959), 1.

28   Roberta Bivins, 'Weighing on Us All? Quantification and Cultural Responses to Obesity in NHS Britain', *History of Science* 58, no. 2 (2020): 216–42.

29   Bivins, 'Weighing on Us All?', 8.

30   'Buns Banned at the Tuckshop', *The Times*, 14 March 1961.

31   'Fallacy of the Fine Fat Baby', *The Times*, 26 September 1962.

32   Phyllis M. Gibbons, 'An Approach to the Treatment of Overweight Adolescents', in *Public Health in Croydon 1965*, ed. S. L. Wright (Croydon: Public Health Department, 1965), 84.

33   Bivins, 'Weighing on Us All?', 11.

34   Bivins, 'Weighing on Us All?', 9.

35   'Alarming Increase in Child Obesity', *The Times*, 5 January 2001.

36   Bivins, 'Weighing on Us All?', 24–5.

37   Bivins, 'Weighing on Us All?', 26.

38   Jan van Eys, ed., *The Normally Sick Child* (Baltimore: University Park Press, 1979), 24.

39 David Wright, '"Childlike in His Innocence": Lay Attitudes to 'Idiots' and 'Imbeciles' in Victorian England', in *From Idiocy to Mental Deficiency: Historical Perspectives on People with Learning Disabilities*, ed. David Wright and Anne Digby (New York: Routledge, 1996), 121.

40 Simon Jarrett, *Those They Called Idiots: The Idea of the Disabled Mind from 1700 to the Present Day* (London: Reaktion, 2020).

41 David Wright, *Mental Disability in Victorian England: The Earlswood Asylum, 1847–1901* (Oxford: Clarendon Press, 2001), 122.

42 Wright, *Mental Disability*, 125.

43 J. Langdon H. Down, 'Observations on an Ethnic Classification of Idiots', *Journal of Mental Science* 13, no. 61 (April 1867): 121–3.

44 Down, 'Observations'.

45 Wright, *Mental Disability*, 125.

46 Although, oddly, it was not free to everyone until 1891. June Purvis, *Hard Lessons: The Lives and Education of Working-Class Women in Nineteenth-Century England* (Cambridge: Polity Press, 1989).

47 Joan Burstyn, *Victorian Education and the Ideal of Womanhood* (New Brunswick, NJ: Rutgers University Press, 1984), 40.

48 Max Roser and Esteban Ortiz-Ospina, 'Literacy' (Oxford: Our World in Data, 2016), ourworldindata.org/literacy.

49 Stephen Jay Gould, *The Mismeasure of Man* (Harmondsworth: Penguin, 1984), 152–3.

50 Darwin to Francis Galton, 23 December [1869] (Cambridge: Darwin Correspondence Project, 2020), accessed 13 January 2022, www.darwinproject.ac.uk/letter/?docId=letters/DCP-LETT-7032.xml.

51 Francis Galton, *Hereditary Genius, an Inquiry into Its Laws and Consequences*, 2nd edn (London: Macmillan, 1914), 29–32.

52 Alfred Binet and Théodore Simon, *The Development of Intelligence in Children (the Binet–Simon Scale)*, trans. Elizabeth S. Kite (Baltimore: Williams & Wilkins, 1916), 7–9.

53 Binet and Simon, *Development of Intelligence*, 46.

54 Gould, *Mismeasure of Man*, 150.

55 Gould, *Mismeasure of Man*, 191.

56 James R. Flynn, 'Massive IQ Gains in 14 Nations: What IQ Tests Really Measure', *Psychological Bulletin* 101, no. 2 (1987): 171–91; James R. Flynn, 'The Mean IQ of Americans: Massive Gains 1932 to 1978', *Psychological Bulletin* 95, no. 1 (1984): 29–51.

57 Richard J. Herrnstein and Charles A. Murray, *The Bell Curve: Intelligence and Class Structure in American Life* (New York: Simon & Schuster, 1994), 298.

58 Ulric Neisser et al., 'Intelligence: Knowns and Unknowns', *American Psychologist* 51, no. 2 (1996): 86.

59 Kathleen W. Jones, *Taming the Troublesome Child: American Families, Child Guidance, and the Limits of Psychiatric Authority* (Cambridge, MA: Harvard University Press, 1999), 1.

60 G. Fielding Blandford, 'Prevention of Insanity (Prophylaxis)', in *Dictionary of Psychological Medicine*, ed. Daniel Hack Tuke, vol. 2 (London: J. & A. Churchill, 1892), 997–8.

61 Frank Wedekind, *Spring Awakening*, trans. Edward Bond (London: Eyre Methuen, 1980), 50.

62 Jones, *Taming the Troublesome Child*, 33.

63 Jones, *Taming the Troublesome Child*, 34.

64 Jane Addams, *The Spirit of Youth and the City Streets* (New York: Macmillan, 1920), 161.

65 Sophonisba Preston Breckinridge and Edith Abbott, *The Delinquent Child and the Home: A Study of the Delinquent Wards of the Juvenile Court of Chicago* (New York: Survey Associates, 1916), 113.

66 Breckinridge and Abbott, *Delinquent Child*, 87.

67 Breckinridge and Abbott, *Delinquent Child*, 83.

68 Alice Smuts and Robert W. Smuts, *Science in the Service of Children, 1893–1935* (New Haven and London: Yale University Press, 2006), 106.

69 William Healy, *The Individual Delinquent: A Text-Book of Diagnosis and Prognosis for all Concerned in Understanding Offenders* (Boston: Little, Brown and Company, 1915), 352.

70 Healy, *Individual Delinquent*, 353.

71 Smuts and Smuts, *Science*, 3.

72 Jones, *Taming the Troublesome Child*, 239.

73 Katie Wright, 'Inventing the "Normal" Child: Psychology, Delinquency, and the Promise of Early Intervention', *History of the Human Sciences* 30, no. 5 (2017): 54.

74 John Bowlby and James Robertson, 'A Two-Year-Old Goes to Hospital', *Proceedings of the Royal Society of Medicine* 46 (1953): 425.

75 Bowlby and Robertson, 'A Two-Year-Old', 426.

76 Bican Polat, 'Before Attachment Theory: Separation Research at the Tavistock Clinic, 1948–1956', *Journal of the History of the Behavioral Sciences* 53, no. 1 (2017): 59.

77 Polat, 'Before Attachment Theory', 61–2.

78 John Bowlby, 'Some Pathological Processes Set in Train by Early Mother–Child Separation', *Journal of Mental Science* 99, no. 415 (1953): 270.

79 Bowlby, 'Some Pathological Processes', 270.

80 Polat, 'Before Attachment Theory', 64.

81 Stephen J. Suomi, Frank C. P. van der Horst, and René van der Veer, 'Rigorous Experiments on Monkey Love: An Account of Harry F. Harlow's Role in the History of Attachment Theory', *Integrative Psychological and Behavioral Science* 42, no. 4 (1 December 2008): 362.

82 Harry F. Harlow, 'The Nature of Love', *American Psychologist* 13, no. 12 (December 1958): 685.

83 *Dr Benjamin Spock's Pocket Book of Baby and Child Care* (New York: Pocket Books, 1953), 270.

84 Spock, *Baby and Child Care*, 220.

85 Illingworth, *The Normal Child*, 216–19.
86 Matthew Smith, *Hyperactive: The Controversial History of ADHD* (London: Reaktion, 2012), 64.
87 Michael E. Staub, *The Mismeasure of Minds: Debating Race and Intelligence Between Brown and The Bell Curve* (Chapel Hill: University of North Carolina Press, 2018), 57.
88 Smith, *Hyperactive*, 52.
89 Smith, *Hyperactive*, 54–5.
90 Staub, *Mismeasure*, 59; 71.
91 Bernard Coard, *How the West Indian Child Is Made Educationally Sub-Normal in the British School System* (London: New Beacon, 1971); Bernard Coard, 'Why I Wrote the "ESN Book"', *Guardian*, 5 February 2005.
92 Staub, *Mismeasure*, 76.
93 Allen Frances and Bernard J. Carroll, 'Keith Conners', *BMJ* 358 (6 July 2017).
94 Tyler Page, *Raised on Ritalin: A Personal Story of ADHD, Medication, and Modern Psychiatry* (Minneapolis: Dementian Comics, 2016), 15.

7 Is Society Normal?

1 Caroline Davies, Pamela Duncan, and Niamh McIntyre, 'UK Coronavirus Deaths Rise by 181 as Confirmed Cases near 15,000', *Guardian*, 27 March 2020. The number of deaths for this period reported on the UK government website is now considerably higher, as it includes those outside hospitals.
2 Margaret Atwood, *The Handmaid's Tale* (London: Vintage, 1996).
3 Arthur Conan Doyle, *The Sign of Four* (Harmondsworth: Penguin, 1982), 22.
4 Conan Doyle, *The Sign of Four*, 99.
5 The Eeyore of Victorian science, as historian James Moore calls him, which sums Spencer up quite nicely. James R. Moore, 'Herbert Spencer's Henchmen: The Evolution of Protestant Liberals in Late Nineteenth-Century America', in *Darwinism and Divinity: Essays on Evolution and Religious Belief*, ed. John R. Durant (Oxford: Blackwell, 1985), 85.
6 Herbert Spencer, *Social Statics; or the Conditions Essential to Human Happiness Specified, and the First of Them Developed* (London: Williams and Norgate, 1868), 493.
7 For more details, see George W. Stocking, *Victorian Anthropology* (New York: Free Press, 1987).
8 Edward B. Tylor, 'Primitive Society (Part I)', *Contemporary Review* 21 (1872): 716.
9 Charles Darwin, *The Descent of Man, and Selection in Relation to Sex*, vol. 1 (London: John Murray, 1871), 158–67.
10 Tylor, 'Primitive Society (Part I)', 716.
11 Arvind Verma, 'Consolidation of the Raj: Notes from a Police Station in British India, 1865–1928', in *Crime, Gender, and Sexuality in Criminal*

Prosecutions, ed. Louis A. Knafla, Criminal Justice History 17 (Westport, CT: Greenwood Press, 2002), 124.

12 Laurence W. Preston, 'A Right to Exist: Eunuchs and the State in Nineteenth-Century India', *Modern Asian Studies* 21, no. 2 (1987): 372.

13 Quoted in Preston, 'Right to Exist', 385.

14 Conan Doyle, *The Sign of Four*, 115.

15 Conan Doyle, *The Sign of Four*, 136.

16 Tylor, 'Primitive Society (Part I)', 717.

17 Sarah E. Igo, *The Averaged American: Surveys, Citizens, and the Making of a Mass Public* (Cambridge, MA: Harvard University Press, 2008), 69.

18 Émile Durkheim, *The Rules of Sociological Method*, ed. George E. G. Catlin, trans. Sarah A. Solovay and John H. Mueller (New York: Free Press, 1966), 74.

19 Helen Merrell Lynd and Robert S. Lynd, *Middletown: A Study in Contemporary American Culture* (New York: Harcourt, Brace and Company, 1929), 4.

20 Igo, *Averaged American*, 70.

21 Lynd and Lynd, *Middletown*, 9.

22 Igo, *Averaged American*, 87.

23 Igo, *Averaged American*, 58.

24 Lynd and Lynd, *Middletown*, 8; Igo, *Averaged American*, 56. Igo puts the figure of white American-born at a slightly lower – but still unusual – 88 per cent.

25 Igo, *Averaged American*, 57.

26 Lynd and Lynd, *Middletown*, 482–3; Igo, *Averaged American*, 59.

27 Igo, *Averaged American*, 59.

28 Lynd and Lynd, *Middletown*, 24.

29 Lynd and Lynd, *Middletown*, 74–5.

30 Lynd and Lynd, *Middletown*, 27.

31 Igo, *Averaged American*, 94.

32 See Anna G. Creadick, *Perfectly Average: The Pursuit of Normality in Postwar America* (Amherst and Boston: University of Massachusetts Press, 2010), 48.

33 Clark Wright Heath, *What People Are: A Study of Normal Young Men* (Cambridge, MA: Harvard University Press, 1946).

34 Creadick, *Perfectly Average*, 58.

35 Heath, *What People Are*, 3. Emphasis in the original.

36 Earnest Albert Hooton, *'Young Man, You Are Normal': Findings from a Study of Students* (New York: Putnam, 1945), 186.

37 Heath, *What People Are*, 5.

38 Hooton, *'Young Man, You Are Normal'*, 209.

39 Clifford Geertz, '"From the Native's Point of View": On the Nature of Anthropological Understanding', *Bulletin of the American Academy of Arts and Sciences* 28, no. 1 (October 1974): 31.

40 Stanley Milgram, *Obedience to Authority: An Experimental View* (New York: Harper & Row, 1974), 29.

41 Milgram, *Obedience to Authority*, 79–81.

42   Ian Nicholson, '"Shocking" Masculinity: Stanley Milgram, "Obedience to Authority", and the "Crisis of Manhood" in Cold War America', *Isis* 102, no. 2 (2011): 262.

43   Martin Gansberg, '37 Who Saw Murder Didn't Call the Police', *The New York Times*, 27 March 1964, 1.

44   A. M. Rosenthal, *Thirty-Eight Witnesses: The Kitty Genovese Case* (Berkeley and London: University of California Press, 1999).

45   Marcia M. Gallo, *'No One Helped': Kitty Genovese, New York City, and the Myth of Urban Apathy* (Ithaca, NY: Cornell University Press, 2015), 34.

46   Émile Durkheim, *Suicide: A Study in Sociology*, ed. George Simpson, trans. John A. Spaulding and George Simpson (London and New York: Routledge, 2002), 332.

47   Kevin O'Keefe, *The Average American: The Extraordinary Search for the Nation's Most Ordinary Citizen* (New York: Public Affairs, 2005), 4.

Epilogue: Beyond the Normal

1   For the full story of this erasure, see Marcia M. Gallo, *'No One Helped': Kitty Genovese, New York City, and the Myth of Urban Apathy* (Ithaca, NY: Cornell University Press, 2015).

2   Adolphe Quetelet, *A Treatise on Man and the Development of His Faculties*, trans. Robert Knox (Edinburgh: W. & R. Chambers, 1842), 8.

INDEX

Page numbers in *italics* refer to illustrations